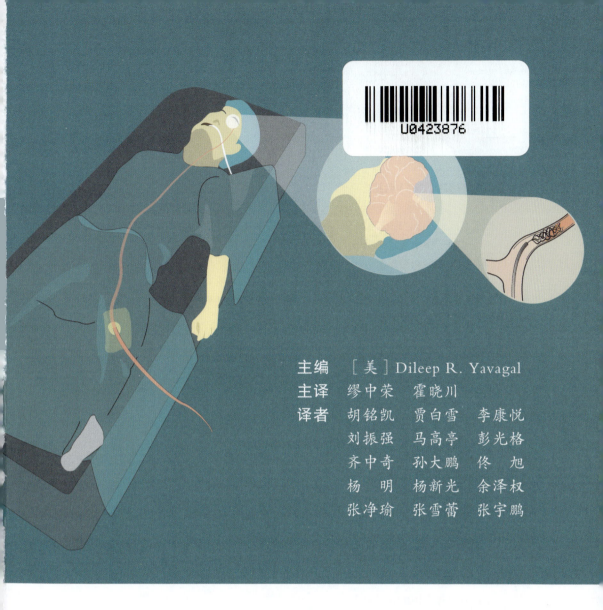

主编 [美] Dileep R. Yavagal
主译 缪中荣　霍晓川
译者 胡铭凯　贾白雪　李康悦
　　　刘振强　马高亭　彭光格
　　　齐中奇　孙大鹏　佟　旭
　　　杨　明　杨新光　余泽权
　　　张净瑜　张雪蕾　张宇鹏

急性卒中机械取栓：现状与经验

卒中政策因地制宜，先进经验全球共享！

电子工业出版社
Publishing House of Electronics Industry
北京·BEIJING

未经许可，不得以任何方式复制或抄袭本书之部分或全部内容。
版权所有，侵权必究。

版权贸易合同登记号　图字：01-2021-3816

图书在版编目（CIP）数据

急性卒中机械取栓：现状与经验 /（美）迪里普·R. 亚瓦加尔（Dileep R. Yavagal）主编；缪中荣，霍晓川主译. —北京：电子工业出版社，2021.7
ISBN 978-7-121-41533-3

Ⅰ.①急… Ⅱ.①迪…②缪…③霍… Ⅲ.①急性病–脑缺血–血栓栓塞–治疗 Ⅳ.①R743.310.5

中国版本图书馆CIP数据核字（2021）第128844号

责任编辑：王梦华
印　　刷：中国电影出版社印刷厂
装　　订：中国电影出版社印刷厂
出版发行：电子工业出版社
　　　　　北京市海淀区万寿路173信箱　邮编：100036
开　　本：720×1000　1/16　印张：7.5　字数：100千字
版　　次：2021年7月第1版
印　　次：2021年7月第2次印刷
定　　价：80.00元

凡所购买电子工业出版社图书有缺损问题，请向购买书店调换。若书店售缺，请与本社发行部联系，联系及邮购电话：（010）88254888，88258888。
质量投诉请发邮件至zlts@phei.com.cn，盗版侵权举报请发邮件到dbqq@phei.com.cn。
本书咨询联系方式：QQ 375096420。

Mission Thrombectomy 2020（MT 2020）

　　MT 2020 是一个致力于通过公共卫生健康政策推广动脉取栓、分享卒中管理先进经验的非营利性全球组织。无论是在哪个国家、患者是多大年龄（主要是在 50 岁以上），卒中都对健康、经济及社会等造成了沉重的负担。2015 年"五大研究"的阳性结果发表以后，急诊取栓已经成为急性大动脉闭塞导致的严重卒中的标准治疗方法。在卒中急性期即 24 小时之内，给予动脉取栓或在时间窗内联合静脉溶栓，是目前挽救缺血半暗带最为有效的治疗策略；而且该治疗方法已证实在不同经济发展水平的国家均具有较高的成本效益比。MT 2020 最早由血管与介入神经病学学会（Society of Vascular and Interventional Neurology，SVIN）在 2016 年策划发起，目前已经成为一个跨学科、多经济体的组织，致力于更加广泛地推广动脉取栓技术，并基于科学证据来影响公共健康政策，使其惠及更多的卒中人群。

免责声明

本报告中的相关作者对所提供的诊疗建议、研究发现及最终结论等数据的准确性负责。但本报告不作为相关的标准和规则。

本报告由血管与介入神经病学学会（SVIN）提供。

缩写表

AC：Anterior Circulation，前循环
AHA：American Heart Association，美国心脏学会
AIS：Acute Ischemic Stroke，急性缺血性卒中
APTT：Activated Partial Thromboplastin Time，活化部分凝血活酶时间
ASA：American Stroke Association，美国卒中学会
BA：Basilar Artery，基底动脉
BP：Blood Pressure，血压
CT：Computed Tomography，计算机断层扫描
CTA：Computed Tomography Angiography，CT血管成像
DALY：Disability-Adjusted Life Years，残疾调整生命年
EKG：Electrocardiogram，心电图
EMS：Emergency Medical Services，急救医疗服务
FDA：Food and Drug Administration，美国食品和药物管理局
GBD：Global Burden of Disease，全球疾病负担
HS：Hemorrhagic Stroke，出血性卒中
ICA：Internal Carotid Artery，颈内动脉
ICH：Intracranial Hemorrhage，颅内出血
IECR：Incremental Cost-Effectiveness Ratio，增量成本-效果比
INR：International Normalized Ratio，国际标准化比率

IV：Intravenous，静脉注射
IVT：Intravenous Thrombolysis，静脉溶栓
LMWH：Low Molecular Weight Heparins，低分子量肝素
LVO：Large Vessel Occlusion，大血管闭塞
M1：Proximal Middle Cerebral Artery，大脑中动脉近端
M2：Distal Middle Cerebral Artery，大脑中动脉远端
MRI：Magnetic Resonance Imaging，磁共振成像
mRS：Modified Rankin Scale Score，改良Rankin量表评分
MT：Mechanical Thrombectomy，机械取栓
NIH：National Institutes of Health，美国国立卫生研究院
NIHSS：National Institutes of Health Stroke Scale，美国国立卫生研究院卒中量表
PT：Prothrombin Time，血浆凝血酶原时间
QALY：Quality Adjusted Life Year，质量调整生命年
QOL：Quality of Life，生活质量
RCT：Randomized Controlled Trial，随机对照试验
rt-PA：Recombinant Tissue Plasminogen Activator，重组组织型纤溶酶原激活物
SDI：Socio-Demographic Index，社会-人口统计指数
SVIN：Society of Vascular and Interventional Neurologists，血管与介入神经病学学会
TIA：Transient Ischemic Attack，短暂性脑缺血发作
t-PA：Tissue Plasminogen Activator，组织型纤溶酶原激活物
TSC：Thrombectomy Systems of Care，取栓中心
US：United States，美国

目 录

摘 要 …………………………………………… 1

背 景 …………………………………………… 5
1. 什么是"中风"或"卒中"？……………………… 5
2. 什么是大血管闭塞（LVO）卒中？……………… 6
3. 目前有哪些治疗手段？……………………………… 6
4. MT：新的标准治疗 ………………………………… 8

大血管闭塞卒中治疗的全球差距 10

1. 卒中与大血管闭塞卒中的发生率：全球视角 10
2. 有效治疗 LVO 卒中的挑战 12

大血管闭塞卒中治疗的革命性飞跃 15

1. MT 成为标准治疗 15
2. MT 的全球成本效益 16
3. LVO 卒中治疗时建议的急救措施 22

如何在您的区域实施 MT 26

1. MT 的社区宣教 26
2. MT 培训计划 27
3. 在您的社区建立取栓系统 28
4. 改善 MT 的院间转诊 30

给政策制定者的建议 33

1. 给政策制定者的关键建议 33

2. 患者诊疗路径的推荐步骤 ·· 34

关于作者 ··· 36

附　录 ··· 37
　　A. 机械取栓治疗急性卒中的文献综述和具体科学证据 ············ 37
　　B. 团队培训原则 ··· 67
　　C. 基本的/主要的预防原则 ··· 68
　　D. 急诊处理原则 ··· 70
　　E. 以医院为中心的急性卒中管理原则 ································· 70
　　F. 二级预防及急性期后管理原则 ·· 74
　　G. 卒中康复原则 ··· 78
　　H. 姑息治疗及临终关怀原则 ··· 83
　　I. 持续治疗改进原则 ·· 84

参考文献 ··· 86

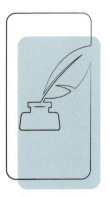

摘 要

在全世界范围内,卒中是首要致残和次要致死原因[1-5]。虽然其他疾病影响患者的时间要多数个月,但是卒中导致的损伤非常迅速:每分钟可造成 200 万神经元凋亡,每小时可造成大脑衰老 3.6 岁,进而可能导致患者终身瘫痪[6]。近年来,唯一可改善预后的溶栓药物能够使患者部分获益,但是仍有约 2/3 的患者遗留有神经功能障碍[7-8],病死率也高达 25%[9-13]。然而,2015 年一项微创手术治疗被证明有效——机械取栓(MT)——使用导管通过腿部的大血管进入大脑,然后将血栓取出[10,14-18]。这项技术与心血管病介入专家开通冠状动脉的操作类似。

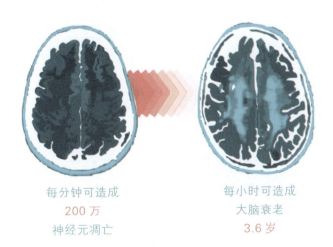

每分钟可造成
200 万
神经元凋亡

每小时可造成
大脑衰老
3.6 岁

急性卒中机械取栓：现状与经验

只要救治时间及时，MT 操作能够将 90% 卒中患者的血栓取出，显著降低神经功能障碍的发生概率[19]。这项技术可以转化卒中诊疗方式，从而有机会挽救成千上万的卒中患者；但前提是，无论何时何地发生卒中，患者所就诊的医院都有能力开展此项治疗。在大多数大血管闭塞（LVO）而导致最严重、最致命的卒中患者中，医生可使用 MT 技术将血栓完全取出[19]，每例患者后续治疗费用将减少 23 000 美元（1 美元 ≈ 6.58 元）[20]，并能成倍降低造成永久性神经功能损伤的概率[24]。虽然 MT 对患者本身和医疗保健系统长期节省支出有诸多好处，但目前仅有约 2000 个取栓中心（TSC）在开展 MT 治疗。其中 900 个在美国，其余的分布于英国、澳大利亚、巴西、日本、法国、德国和西班牙[21]，这说明这项挽救生命的卒中救治技术尚未在全球广泛普及[22,23]。尽管 MT 挽救生命的能力远远超过大部分血管介入治疗，但其获益性在全球卒中负担较重的人群中并不是平均分布的。

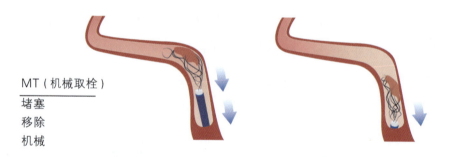

MT（机械取栓）
堵塞
移除
机械

越早治疗获益越大，因此推广 MT 最大的限制因素是如何使患者尽快接受治疗[9,25,26]。急救人员已经创造出把患者从边远地区空运或者转运至 TSC 的创新方法，但是绝大部分患者仍然地处偏远，难以在有效的时间窗内到达 TSC[27]。由于卒中风险广泛存在，医生在努力改进治疗方法的同时，迫切需要对医疗保健政策系统层面的卒中救治转运方式进行变革，使取栓带来的获益从发达国家的城市中心地区推广至所有地区。如果有能够使取栓技术推广到更广泛人群的政策发布，有新的卒中中心建立，新一代的卒中医生被培训，急诊反应系统可以全球协作，那么就能有数以百万计的生命得到挽救[28]，而且每例患者的残疾护理费用能减少至少 23 000 美元[20]。

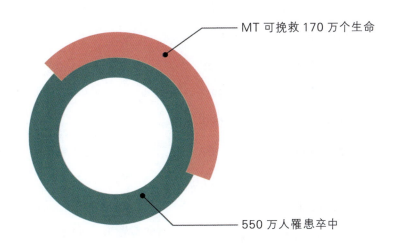

这个问题变得日益凸显，不仅是因为每天有超过 15 000 例患者死于卒中[5]，还因为卒中患者年龄多在 65 岁以上，快速老龄化的人群会显著增加卒中负担[29,30]。事实上，美国心脏协会（AHA）指出，2012 年美国卒中总花费高达 716 亿美元，而 2030 年这项支出会迅速增长至 1831 亿美元[31]。此项开支超过了美国国家卫生研究院（NIH）对医学研究、国防部高级研究工程、美国国家航空航天局、卫生和公众服务部、急诊部门、国土安全、住房和城市发展部的预算总和[31-38]。此外，公众卫生的财政负担会持续增长。建立卒中系统仍然需要时间，但是取栓治疗的有效性已经在 9 项随机对照试验的 17 项研究中的 1077 例患者中得到证实[9,10,13-16,18,26,32,39-40]。这些卒中系统被证实能够显著改善患者预后，每位患者的治疗费用将节省数千美元[33]。如果卒中系统能够建立起来，解决日益增长的卒中负担和卒中所致的残疾负担，我们不仅能挽救生命，还能够显著减少那些无法转

急性卒中机械取栓：现状与经验

运至最佳治疗中心患者的远期治疗费用。

血管与介入神经病学学会（SVIN）引领着介入放射学的进步，其目的是改善全球卒中和脑血管病的临床救治和患者预后。2016年，SVIN启动了"取栓使命2020"，旨在整合全球的力量，于2020年将年取栓量从100 000例增加至202 000例，实现全球范围内卒中相关残疾率的下降，并且挽救数百万患者的生命。为了践行这项使命，SVIN与政府机构、非营利医疗组织和行业领军者合作，提高民众意识，建立财政措施以支持取栓系统的发展。

我们组织了卒中团体的领导者，从取栓装置的发明者和顶级医院的医生和研究者，到全世界卒中系统的建设者，共同参与本报告的编写，不仅为了阐述卒中对社会带来的危害和新型卒中疗法潜在的益处，还提供了一本如何在全世界建立卒中系统的指导手册。我们希望广大医疗团体、医疗健康管理者和公共政策制定者能够使用本报告来指导工作，帮助制定切实有效的治疗方法，从而使深受疾病困扰的患者获益。我们整理了以下材料，来帮助大家为实现这个目标而努力。

这份报告的目标

1. 教育 关于MT治疗卒中的相关教育
2. 建议 建立取栓护理系统的建议
3. 鼓励 鼓励决策者改进MT的实施以减少全球卒中负担

背 景

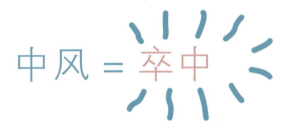

1. 什么是"中风"或"卒中"？

当大脑的主要供血动脉发生阻塞或破裂，导致部分大脑缺乏氧气和营养时，就会发生卒中，俗称中风[34]。当这种脑损伤是由于血管的突然阻塞造成时，即为急性缺血性卒中（AIS）；如果是由血管破裂引起的，则为出血性卒中（HS）。氧气供应减少几分钟后，就有可能造成永久性脑损伤，导致脑细胞死亡，并引起显著的神经系统症状，如突然出现的单侧面部或肢体的麻木无力，伴有神志不清、视物不清、行走困难和严重头痛等[41,35]。

2. 什么是大血管闭塞（LVO）卒中？

大血管闭塞（LVO）卒中，是指由于头颈部 4 条主要脑供血动脉中的任意一条发生闭塞所导致的缺血性卒中[52-59]。LVO 卒中约占 AIS 总人数的 1/3，因其缺血范围大且脑损伤严重[62,63]，因此致死、致残率极高[58,60,61]。闭塞通常是在原有狭窄血管的基础上形成血栓，或因身体其他部位的血栓进入并引起脑动脉栓塞[34]。

3. 目前有哪些治疗手段？

对疑似 AIS 患者的治疗包括以下措施。首先，完成头颅 CT 和 MRI 排除出血性卒中；然后考虑药物溶栓和机械取栓治疗，同时给予一般的支持性治疗。在治疗过程中，实时观察和处理突发的药物不良反应和相关的神经系统并发症。最后，评估此次卒中最有可能的病因，并针对病因制定二级预防方案，预防卒中复发。根据不同医疗机构治疗水平和医疗设备的差异，可以考虑以下任何一种治疗方法。

静脉溶栓（IVT）

静脉溶栓或使用溶栓药物是美国食品和药物管理局（FDA）批准的唯一治疗 AIS 患者的药物治疗方案。静脉溶栓与改善患者的预后相关。虽然一些研究提示，遗传差异、种族和性别可能会影响 IVT 的治疗效果，但目前仅在一些特殊情况下，AIS 患者才对 IVT 反应较差，如高血压（血压升高）和高血糖（血糖水平升高）[68-74]。然而，IVT 治疗 LVO 卒中的作用却十分有限，因为往往 LVO 缺血范围较大和血栓负荷较高。

机械取栓（MT）

MT 是一种微创手术。通过股动脉穿刺，把取栓装置通过血管通路送至血管闭塞的位置，然后穿过闭塞血管，通过取栓的器械把血栓取出，使血管血流得以恢复，从而逆转脑损伤。

MT操作流程：

- 微导管定位：微导管经股动脉（或桡动脉）入路置入血管，通过颈部向上推进到达责任血管闭塞部位。
- 支架输送：利用X线透视指导，将可回收支架（一种可以使LVO再通的细长机械工具）插入微导管。
- 支架定位、释放及回收：将支架穿过血栓，打开支架以支撑血管壁，使血液流动恢复，然后"回收"——即向后拉，从而取出血栓。

IVT联合MT

无论年龄大小和卒中严重程度如何，发病24小时内的LVO-AIS患者接受MT联合IVT，可以显著提高临床预后良好的患者比例[75]。单独应用IVT会受到4.5小时治疗时间窗的限制，且对较大负荷的血栓无治疗效果，使得其对LVO-AIS患者无效[75-77]。因此，联合使用IVT和MT可以互相弥补不足，克服上述限制[76]。

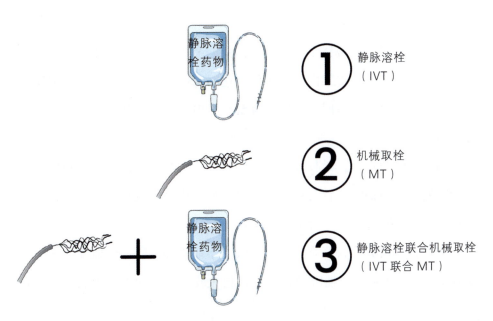

4. MT：新的标准治疗

卒中起病迅速、病情发展及救治流程的时间依赖性强，这些都给治疗带来很大困难。

卒中患者的治疗每延缓1分钟，就会有200万个脑细胞、140亿个神经连接和12公里长的神经纤维受到损伤。总体来看，这些损伤可以使大脑每小时老化3.6岁。因此，AIS患者能否尽早接受治疗至关重要[6]。

IVT的治疗时间窗很短，大多数AIS患者必须在发病4.5小时内接受IVT[151]；同时，IVT的治疗效果取决于血栓的大小，这使得IVT不是治疗LVO-AIS的有效选择[78,79,152-153]。大量研究表明，MT可以使闭塞血管快速恢复血流（再通），改善患者的预后，同时将急性期AIS的治疗时间窗扩大到24小时[9,11,12,15,16,18,26,32]。

MT是一种使用微导管和取栓器械，以机械方式捕获并移除闭塞血管中的血栓的微创介入手术。

MT操作使用的器械根据其作用机制不同可分为两种：可回收支架和抽吸导管。相应地，MT方法包括：①可回收支架取栓；②抽吸导管取栓；③可回收支架联合抽吸导管取栓。

可回收支架取栓装置是由可膨胀扩张的金属网制成的，作用是将血栓完整地取出。可回收支架由输送导管送达闭塞部位。到位后，金属网膨胀扩张，锚定血栓，然后回撤取栓装置至导管内，将导管和取栓装置一起从患者体内取出[80]。

抽吸导管内径大，柔韧性极佳。将导丝置入微导管内引导抽吸导管至血管闭塞处。当抽吸导管与血栓接触时，将血栓分解成更小的碎片，用泵或手动吸引器通过抽吸导管将血栓移除[154]。

在最近的研究中，联合应用可回收支架取栓和抽吸导管取栓显示出一定优势[81]。在美国，抽吸导管的价格相对较低，因此首先尝试抽吸导管取栓。如果失败，则通过抽吸导管置入可回收支架来尝试机械取栓。使用这种顺序或并行的组合，可以实现高达95%的再通率[81]，而单独使用抽吸导管的再通率为78%。

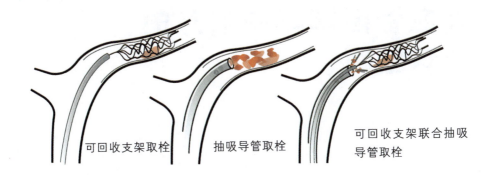

可回收支架取栓　　抽吸导管取栓　　可回收支架联合抽吸导管取栓

大血管闭塞卒中治疗的全球差距

1. 卒中与大血管闭塞卒中的发生率：全球视角

卒中的人口统计资料

目前，卒中是全球第二大死亡原因和致残的主要原因[51,82]。2010年，全球 AIS 的发病人口估计为 1160 万人；63% 的 AIS 和 80% 的 HS 发生在中低收入国家[84]。2016年，全球卒中发病人口为 1370 万，导致 550 万人死亡[3]。在美国，年龄在 35~44 岁成年人卒中的发病率为每年 30~120 / 10 万人，而年龄在 65~74 岁成年人卒中的发病率为每年 670~970 / 10 万人[107,108]。与年轻卒中患者相比，年龄的增加还伴随着更高的死亡率和生活质量（QOL）的下降[109-114]。

根据一项全球疾病负担（GBD）的研究，2016年全球25岁或以上年龄的人群，卒中的终身风险估计接近 25%，男性和女性的发病率几乎相等[126]。

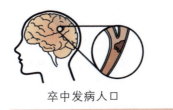
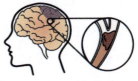

卒中发病人口　　　　　　　LVO 发病人口

1370 万　　　　　　　　　510 万

LVO 的发生率——跨人口统计数据

在所有与卒中相关的死亡中，约有一半归因于 AIS[5]。LVO 与更差的预后明显相关[128]，使 6 个月内死亡的概率增加 4.5 倍[60]。据报道，由 LVO 引起的 AIS（AIS-LVO）占 11%~46%[57,59,60,129,131]。

美国

在美国，平均每 40 秒就有一个人发生卒中[96,97]。卒中是第五大死因，每年发病人数约为 80 万，有超过 14.6 万人死亡（19 人中有 1 人死亡），是导致严重残疾的主要原因，使得许多人长期残疾和无法工作[97]。

由 LVO 引起的 AIS 估计每年发生率为 24/10 万人，相当于每年有将近 8 万例 LVO 卒中[59]。

中国

在中国，卒中是最主要的死亡原因，占所有死亡人数的 22.45%[131]。事实上，中国有 700 多万人经历过卒中，其中 65% 是 AIS[134]。此外，所有 AIS 中有 35%~40% 是由 LVO 引起的[131]。

日本

2017 年，卒中是日本的第三大死因[136]，每年卒中发病率为 142.9/10 万人。AIS 的发病率为 91.3/10 万人/年[137]。

中东地区：沙特阿拉伯

每年卒中发生率为 22.7~250 / 10 万人。男性比女性更常见，其平均发病年龄为 60~70 岁。AIS 是最常见的卒中类型，而高血压和糖尿病是最常见的卒中危险因素[138]。

印度

在过去的 20 年中，印度的卒中累积发病率为每年 105~152 / 10 万人。与全球的估计数相比，其卒中发生率高于高收入国家[146-148]。

2. 有效治疗 LVO 卒中的挑战

静脉溶栓（IVT）不适用于 LVO 卒中

唯一被批准用于治疗 AIS 的药物是静脉溶栓药物；然而，这些药物对 LVO 引起的 AIS 患者无效，因为 LVO 患者的血栓负荷量大，尤其是当血栓长度超过 8mm 时[165]。此外，IVT 需要在症状出现后 4.5 小时的狭窄时间窗内进行，这使得超过 85% 的患者失去了溶栓资格[157-160]。

对于 LVO 卒中，MT 是标准的治疗方法，因为它可以机械地清除大块阻塞的血栓，并且可以在卒中症状出现后长达 24 小时内进行[157-160]。

需要增加 MT 数量

MT 通常由神经介入专家进行。神经介入专业是神经放射学的一个亚专业，通过血管内入路，将各种器械输送到先前确定的病灶处实施微创手术。据估计，美国每年每 10 万人中有 3 人接受 MT，每年有 1 万例 MT[59,61]。因此，MT 数量远远低于 LVO 卒中的发生率，这表明需要进一步利用取栓技术，增加取栓数量。

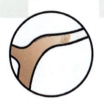 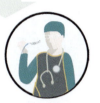

LVO 发生率　　　　MT 需求　　　　神经介入专家

静脉注射 rt-PA 治疗 AIS 的禁忌证
1. 出现卒中症状超过 4.5 小时
2. 在过去 3 个月内有卒中或严重头部外伤病史
3. 有颅内出血史
4. 症状提示蛛网膜下腔出血
5. 长期血压升高（收缩压 ≥ 185mmHg 或舒张压 ≥ 110mmHg）
6. 低血糖（血糖 < 1.7mmol/L）或 PT > 15 秒
7. 48 小时内使用过肝素，并伴有 APTT 值异常升高
8. 在过去 7 天内在不可压迫的部位进行了动脉穿刺
9. 在 21 天内有消化道出血病史
10. 在 14 天内曾接受重大手术、颅内或脊柱内手术
11. 既往有动脉瘤、动静脉畸形或颅内肿瘤病史
12. 目前正在使用直接凝血酶抑制剂或 Xa 因子抑制剂，并伴有各种实验室检查异常（如 APTT、INR<ECT、TT 或 Xa 因子活性检测等）
13. CT 上可见不可逆的早期缺血改变超过大脑中动脉供血区的 1/3，或存在颅内出血

　　随着老龄化人口的增长，这些数字预计还会增加。LVO 卒中发病率的增加预计会出现对神经介入专家、MT 操作和设备以及具备 MT 能力的医院的需求增加[171]。

　　根据权威的健康数据库，目前美国有 900 家 MT 治疗中心[172]。美国的卒中治疗市场增长迅速，主要是由于 AIS 器械市场的扩大，预计到 2026 年，其总量将翻番[172]。美国的卒中干预模式正在向专业的大容量卒中中心转型，并鼓励患者直接绕行至取栓中心，以便更及时地开始治疗[173]。取栓中心的认证过程既耗时又昂贵，这限制了这些中心的发展；而且农村 / 人

急性卒中机械取栓：现状与经验

口稀少地区的服务仍然不足，因为在人口不足的地区建立新设施往往是不合理的。然而，由于 AIS 器械和 MT 手术费用在美国是全额报销的，因此卒中治疗量预计在未来 10 年将大幅增加。但是，鉴于医疗卫生系统主要是自费和有限的保险报销，支持在低收入和中等收入国家设立取栓中心仍具挑战性。

强烈建议这些国家的政策制定者和政府官员给予干预，加快推广 MT，以减轻仅凭 IVT 无法解决的 LVO-AIS 所带来的日益增加的负担。

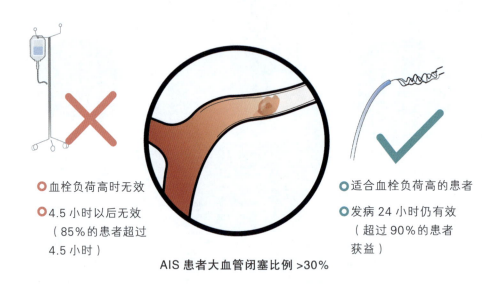

- 血栓负荷高时无效
- 4.5 小时以后无效（85% 的患者超过 4.5 小时）

AIS 患者大血管闭塞比例 >30%

- 适合血栓负荷高的患者
- 发病 24 小时仍有效（超过 90% 的患者获益）

大血管闭塞卒中治疗的革命性飞跃

1. MT 成为标准治疗

在过去的 20 年里,随着卒中循证医学的发展,卒中治疗发生了显著的变化,增加了卒中患者获得优先治疗的概率,并改善了卒中的急救管理[191-200]。MT 的出现被认为是 LVO 卒中治疗的突破性进展。从脑动脉中使用机械材料取出血栓,给卒中患者带来了更好的预后,包括更快速、更显著的功能独立性的结局。

许多临床试验已经证明 MT 可以带来更好的临床预后,从而使其被广泛应用。事实上,MT 的手术量在 3 年内翻了 1 倍,预计每年将以 25% 的速度增长,到 2025 年将达到 202 020 例。2018 年《ASA 指南》推荐 LVO 卒中患者进行急诊 MT[199]。

MT 与其他治疗方式相比有许多优势[202-204],包括:

(1)提高了血管再通率,降低了远期残疾率[55]。

(2)与 IVT 相比,MT 将治疗时间窗扩展到卒中发病后 24 小时。IVT 受限于 4.5 小时的静脉溶栓时间窗,因此只有较少的 AIS 患者能接受

IVT[26]。

（3）可取出IVT无效的血栓，例如质地较硬并含有胆固醇结晶的陈旧性血栓或大血栓。

2. MT的全球成本效益

卒中治疗能否达到最佳疗效，具有时间敏感性，更短的发病 – 治疗时间将会有更高概率获得功能改善、血流恢复和脑组织挽救[9,10,14-18,26]。预后的改善与减轻经济负担密切相关。实际上，在6小时内对AIS进行快速治疗可缩短3~7天的住院时间和1~5个月的康复周期。因此，与更长的治疗时间（＞6小时）或未再通相比，能降低5000~50 000美元的费用[205]。

北美

机械血栓切除术快速再通的成本效益

	发病 – 再通时间		
	≤6小时	＞6小时	未再通
住院天数	9.8 ± 5.8	13.2 ± 8.1	16.7 ± 19.3
康复期（天）	87.2 ± 136.4	133.7 ± 152.4	224 ± 130.3
1年康复费用	\$16 024 ± 12 320	\$21 002 ± 15 504	\$29 382 ± 17 403
功能独立	70%	40%	6%
家庭式出院	72%	50%	21%
死亡	10%	16%	43%
成本效益比（与未再通相比）	（\$27 829 /QALY）	（\$24 647 / QALY）	基线

数据来源于2019年Jeong等的回顾性成本效益分析[155]

美国

在美国，AIS带来了很高的经济负担，特别是对于卒中后残疾的出院患者，其费用是非残疾患者的两倍以上（\$120753 *vs* \$54580）[206]。尽管联合治疗（MT

联合 IVT）的初始住院费用（$17 183）比标准治疗（IVT）更高，但由于残疾的大幅减少以及整体生活质量的改善，每位患者一生可节省 $23 203。此外，它还与卒中后康复和护理（90 天费用）和终身成本降低有关[20]。

美国机械血栓切除术成本效益

	联合治疗	标准治疗	P 值	差值
住院费用指数[a]	9.8 ± 5.8	13.2 ± 8.1	<0.001	$17 183
90 天费用[b]	$11 270	$16 174	0.014	($4904)
QRAL[c]	0.131	0.105	0.005	0023
预计 QRAL[d]	6.79	5.05	–	1.74
预计寿命卒中相关费用	$215 781	$238 984	–	$23 203

数据来源于 2017 年 Shireman 等与 SWIFT PRIME 同期开展的前瞻性成本效益研究[20]，a: 初始住院期间的费用；b: 出院至 90 天的费用；c: 生活质量年；d: 预计生活质量年

加拿大

加拿大 AIS 的年平均费用为 28 亿美元，每位患者的平均成本为 $75 353 / 年[209]。与美国的数据类似，卒中相关残疾患者的年平均费用是非残疾患者的两倍以上（$ 107 883 vs $ 48 339）[209]。预计 AIS 的联合治疗每年会为加拿大医疗系统节省 $321334[211]。

欧洲

欧洲机械血栓切除术成本效益

	联合治疗	标准治疗	差值
费用	$6 475 728	$5 249 473	$12 262 551
QRAL	4.842	3.790	1.052
净收益			
下限	$9 503 135	$7 256 379	–
上限	$17 492 566	$13 509 306	–

数据来源于 2015 年 Ganesalingam 等的基于成本效用模型的机械血栓切除术分析[163]。费用基于 2013—2014 年的价格。净收益按 QRAL 的支付意愿的下限和上限计算，在英国分别为 $33 000（£20 000）和 $49500（£30 000）

英国

在英国也有类似情况，联合治疗比标准治疗的初始住院费用更高（$64 757.28 vs $52 494.73）[212]。联合治疗在短期内（90天）不具有成本效益，但预计在20年内[163]和整个生命周期内具有成本效益[214]，如果全面实施，则预计5年内的价值为13亿英镑（17亿美元）[214]。

法国

与美国的结果类似，在法国，联合治疗的初始住院费用比标准治疗高2116美元。然而，卒中后90天获得功能独立的患者数增加了10.9%。每增加一个QALY的预计成本为14 880美元，估计的净收益为2 757美元，这表明了MT在一年时的成本效益[216]。

瑞典

在瑞典，尽管MT增加了干预成本［＋￡9000（$11 779）］，但由于对家庭医疗［－￡13 000（$17 014）］或护理服务（－￡26 000［$34 027］）的依赖性降低，从长远来看可以节省大量费用[218]。

意大利

从意大利国家医疗保健系统（NHS）的角度来看，LVO卒中的联合治疗在卒中后1~3年具有成本效益，从第4年起可节省成本。在卒中后第1年，MT费用比标准治疗费用多€4078.37（$4553.77）［€413 430.81（$14 996.37）vs €49 352.44（$10 442.61）］。在第5年，在与标准治疗相比，联合治疗可节省€3057（$3411）［€431 798（$35 483）vs €434 855（$38 895）］[220]。

意大利机械血栓切除术成本效益

	联合治疗	标准治疗	差值
1 年费用 QALYs ICER	€ 13 430.81 0.55 € 23 990.44	€ 13 430.81 0.55	€ 4078.37 0.17
2 年费用 QALYs ICER	€ 18 096.88 1.08 € 6696.22	€ 15 895.04 0.75	€ 2201.84 0.55
3 年费用 QALYs ICER	€ 22 737.48 1.59 € 798.00	€ 22 353.22 1.11	€ 384.26 0.48
4 年费用 QALYs ICER	€ 2 730 847 2.07	€ 2 867 884 1.44	€ 1370.37 0.63
5 年费用 QALYs ICER	€ 3 179 822 2.52	€ 3 485 490 1.75	€ 3056.68 0.77

数据来源于 2018 年 Ruggeri 等的基于成本效益模型的机械血栓切除术分析[170]。
ICER：增量成本效益比

西班牙

西班牙机械血栓切除术成本效益

	联合治疗	标准治疗	差值
治疗费用	€ 8428.00	€ 1606.00	€ 6822.00
长期管理	€ 105 624.00	€ 157 668.00	€ 52 044.00
成本			
全部 QALYs	7.62	5.11	2.51
寿命年获得	11.708	10.536	1.172

数据来源于 2017 年 Andres-Nogales 等的回顾性成本效益分析[171]

急性卒中机械取栓：现状与经验

从西班牙 NHS 的角度来看，与美国的情况类似，与标准治疗相比，联合治疗的费用较高［€8428.00（美国 $9405）vs €1606.00（美国 $1792）］，但总体费用较低［€123 866（美国 $138 228）］vs €168 244（美国 $187 752）］，净收益为 €119 744（美国 $133 628）[221]。接受联合治疗的患者的结局也得到了改善，延长了 1.17 个寿命年。因此，LVO-AIS 患者的联合治疗成本较低，且比单纯标准治疗更有益[221]。

澳大利亚

澳大利亚机械血栓切除术成本效益

	联合治疗	标准治疗	差值	P 值
住院费用	$29 371	$33 736	($4365)	
住院天数	5	8	(3)	0.04
康复期（天）	0	27	(27)	0.03
QALYs	9.3	4.9	4.4	0.03
效用分数	0.91	0.65	0.26	0.005
DALYs 15 年	5.5	8.9	(3.4)	0.02
预期寿命	15.6	11.2	4.4	0.02

数据来源于 2017 年 Campbell 等的回顾性机械血栓切除术相关的残疾、生活质量、生存和急性期治疗费用分析[11]。

DALY：残疾调整寿命年

在澳大利亚，联合治疗的住院费用较高（$10 666/人），但与标准治疗相比，每例患者一生可节省 8000 多美元[221]。在 90 天内，平衡了医院间运输（平均 $573）和 MT（平均 $10 515）的额外费用后，接受联合治疗患者的平均住院费用低于标准治疗（$15 689 vs $30 569），每位患者平均节省了 $4365（$29 371 vs $33 736）。与接受标准治疗的患者相比，接受 MT 治疗患者的住院时间（5 天 vs 8 天）和康复期（0 vs 27 天）更短，却延长了 4.4 个寿命年[11]。因此，可以预期，联合治疗的增加会减少经济负担[11]。

亚洲

中国

中国机械血栓切除术成本效益

	联合治疗	标准治疗	差值
1 年费用（元） QALYs ICER	77 700 0.405 638 987	27 220 0.326	50 480 0.79
5 年费用（元） QALYs ICER	107 710 1.765 131 689	58 590 1.392	49 120 0.373
6 年费用（元） QALYs ICER	114 170 2.029 113 814	65 230 1.599	48 940 0.43
30 年费用（元） QALYs ICER	167 970 3.773 63 010	117 940 2.979	50 030 0.794

数据来源于 2018 年 Pan 等的回顾性成本效益分析[173]。

在中国，联合治疗在卒中后 5 年被认为不具有成本效益，但在 6 年及以后，被认为具有成本效益[223]。

总结

MT 的成本效益已在全球范围内进行了分析。与标准治疗相比，MT 在更长的时间范围内更具有成本效益。这是因为其可以延长生存时间，提高生存率和生活质量，并减少长期看护（例如护理和康复）。AIS 的卫生经济研究主要来自发达国家，但正在扩展到新的地区，并且费用可能会根据年龄、手术类型和患者基线状况进行分层。

3. LVO 卒中治疗时建议的急救措施

卒中治疗系统要求协调和整合所有救治环节，包括社区教育、预防、紧急医疗服务、卒中救治单元的取栓中心、治疗专家、具备 IVT 和 MT 的能力以及与康复部门的协作等。在全球范围内，高级卒中救治体系的发展具备每年挽救近 200 万人生命的潜力[28]，但这主要取决于患者的及时就诊[187]。由于老龄化和 LVO 卒中发病率的迅速增长，让更多的患者进入取栓中心是近 10 年来主要的公共卫生问题之一。

卒中的治疗是一个复杂的、多步骤的过程，需要及时和准确的诊疗，以增加取得良好预后的可能性。在建设高效的卒中救治系统时，从患者的角度出发，经验十分重要。

大血管闭塞卒中治疗的革命性飞跃

一、患者或目击者电话急救响应

急性卒中救治的第一步是识别 LVO 卒中疾病本身。由于影响较大面积的脑组织，LVO 卒中常会导致更为明显的临床症状。患者可表现为肢体无力，言语不清或者一侧面瘫[230]。这些症状可能很快缓解，或者持续较长一段时间。患者可能会电话求助，或者向他人诉说这些症状，然后由他人电话求助，或者这些症状最初由身边的目击者发现。卒中患者可能无法诉说这些症状，因此旁观者能否发现和识别卒中症状，对患者是否能得到及时充分的救治至关重要。早期识别 LVO 卒中的症状是关键，决定着患者将被转运至可快速进行取栓治疗的取栓中心[230, 231]。一旦怀疑为卒中发作，需要立即呼叫急救医疗服务（emergency medical services，EMS）。

（基于循证医学证据的最佳做法之一是呼叫 EMS，而不是试图转运患者。家属们可能不知道需要将患者转运至哪里，同时也需要通知相应的医院。）

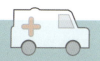

二、急救人员在救护车上的响应

当 EMS 到达后，急救人员应先评估患者，包括询问患者和/或目击者，明确患者症状，导致他们致电 EMS 的事件，以及患者正常的最后时间[192,193]。EMS 可能会进一步询问患者的病史，包括卒中的危险因素，例如高血压、糖尿病、心律失常和患者目前的用药情况。他们也将评估患者的气道、呼吸和血液循环，就像其他危重患者一样[192]。这些初步的综合评估有助于 EMS 专业人员识别 LVO 卒中。EMS 人员还将在患者手臂或手腕建立静脉通路进行输液，如生理盐水和葡萄糖，并协助完成将在医院进行的影像学检查。

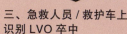

三、急救人员/救护车上识别 LVO 卒中

EMS 人员在检查患者的时候，会使用一些卒中量表，比如面-臂-语音试验（Face Arm Speech Test，FAST）、辛辛那提院前卒中量表（Cincinnati Prehospital Stroke Scale，CPSS）和洛杉矶院前卒中评估量表（Los Angeles Prehospital Stroke Screen，LAPSS）等。这些量表本质上是涵盖患者临床先兆、症状和一些协助诊断 LVO 卒中问题的清单，有助于识别出 LVO 卒中的患者。

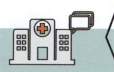

四、急诊室卒中警报

一旦启动卒中急救信号，医生和院内人员将为患者的到院做准备。这使得医院能够启动本院流程，准备必要的药物和 CT 机，在患者到达即刻开始评估。

五、预先通知急诊室

患者被转运至最近的卒中中心。途中，EMS 专业人员应预先通知收治医院，以便院内启动卒中急救信号，并迅速为影像学检查、静脉溶栓和取栓做好准备。

六、急诊室快速通道和紧急影像学评估以及 IVT（如需要）

到达急诊室后，准备就绪的医务人员将得到一份患者病历来了解所有相关信息。这主要是为了排除任何类似卒中症状的其他疾病，如癫痫、偏头痛或低血糖[193]。然后对患者进行神经系统检查，通常包括腱反射，眼球运动，肢体肌力和语言功能等。检查的结果将用于评估症状的严重程度的美国国立卫生研究院卒中量表（NIHSS）评分[195]。在此期间，根据患者的病情需要，可能会给予患者持续心电监护、吸氧、心电图、血液化验、生理盐水静脉补液、胰岛素降血糖和退热药降温治疗[196]。

初步检查之后，患者将行影像学检查。影像学检查在区分 AIS 和 HS 方面至关重要，需根据其结果决定和实施恰当的针对不同卒中类型的治疗方案。中重度卒中患者在接受取栓治疗之前，需行 CT、MRI 或者 CTA 以明确卒中的诊断[193, 196]。

如果影像学结果提示为卒中，下一步应决定治疗方案。许多 AIS 患者接受了 IVT 治疗。IVT 治疗需在发病后 3~4.5 小时内进行[194, 195]。接受 IVT 时间越早，预后越好。因此，发病 60 分钟内行 IVT 治疗是医疗机构的目标[194]。如果 CTA 确诊为 LVO 卒中，则需行 MT 或者 IVT 联合 MT 治疗[195]。

七、取栓团队警报

MT 治疗专门用于救治 LVO 卒中，已接受 IVT 或有适应证但超过静脉溶栓时间窗的患者[194, 196, 197]。发病 6 小时内或者部分发病 6~24 小时的患者可接受取栓治疗[196]。MT 由神经介入医生进行操作。一旦启动卒中信号，神经介入医生就开始进行术前准备，患者准备好后便可立即开始手术。AHA/ASA 发布了 AIS 进行 MT 的筛选标准：发病前功能独立；发病 4.5 小时内接受 IVT；脑组织供血的四大动脉之一的血管闭塞所致的卒中；年龄 ≥ 18 岁；高 NIHSS 评分[194]。

八、腹股沟穿刺

如果患者可行 MT，手术第一步为腹股沟穿刺（或者经手部大血管），这一步需在发病 6 小时内完成[196]。

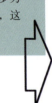

大血管闭塞卒中治疗的革命性飞跃

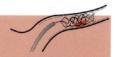

九、LVO 卒中的血栓切除术的过程
　　手术操作包括在腹股沟处的动脉（股动脉）或者手部动脉（桡动脉）置入导管，将导管向上输送经过颈部，直至到达血栓部位。通过 X 线引导成像，将取栓支架和/或抽吸装置送入导管。当支架超过血栓远端后，释放支架，最后回撤移除血栓，或抽出血栓[198]

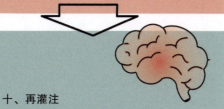

十、再灌注
　　移除血栓可以恢复血管内的血流，并逆转对大脑造成的暂时性损伤。

如何在您的区域实施 MT

1. MT 的社区宣教

医疗专家和公共卫生官员需要制定卒中教育计划，重点关注卒中症状，寻求急诊治疗和可用的卒中系统资源[229]。该计划应该面向社区内的所有人群，以符合经济、社会和伦理的需求[230]。提高对卒中症状的认识，对于寻求及时治疗至关重要[229]。与普通人群相比，社区少数人群对卒中的危险因素和症状的认识度较低。因此，他们很少呼叫 EMS，从而导致必要治疗的延误[231]。延误治疗将会导致治疗效果下降，并使死亡率增加[232]。近几年，随着综合卒中治疗系统的建立，以及公共卒中教育的加强，IVT 和 MT 的例数明显增加。此外，应提高人们对周围可用的急诊调度系统的认识，以缩短卒中发生时间到 EMS 到达的时间间隔[229]。EMS 的激活和卒中患者的转运将提高以下相关情况的比例：更早到达医院（发病到入院时间 ≤ 3 小时）、更快的评估（入院到成像时间 ≤ 25 分钟）、更快的治疗转运（入院到穿刺时间 ≤ 60 分钟）和更多患者符合 MT[223]。

2. MT 培训计划

EMS 培训、评估和管理

卒中治疗的时间窗很短。因此，EMS 专业人员应在快速诊断、评估、管理、治疗、分诊和快速运送卒中患者等方面训练有素并经验丰富[234]。234 名患者预后改善已证实与 EMS 调度员和卒中评估和确诊的现场人员指导患者选择最合适的取栓中心有关[235,236]。

为了使急救医护人员对疑似 LVO 卒中的患者做好准备，EMS 需向接收医院提供到达前的通知。事实上，这将使患者在 3 小时内可接受 IVT 的概率增加、到院 - 影像学检查时间缩短、入院到穿刺时间以及症状出现 - 穿刺时间缩短[244]。此外，基于 EMS 能够识别 LVO 卒中患者，并将患者转运到设备完善的卒中中心，对患者的良好预后至关重要。

培训神经介入医生

MT 的操作医生必须具备相关技术的足够培训的经历和经验，包括基础培训和专业继续教育[245,246]。然而，只有少数医院能给医生提供 MT 培训。因此，建立专门的区域取栓中心十分有必要，以确保医生有足够的 MT 手术量和操作经验[247]。

基线培训和资格

住院医师培训内容包括：在有资质认证的神经放射科医生、神经内科医生或神经外科医生的指导下，AIS 的诊断和管理，CTA 和其他神经影像学的读片，最终获得技术专长。培训临结束时，他们必须获得该领域的资质认证。然后，在高容量的中心，以及神经介入医生的监督下接受 AIS 的神经介入放射学专科培训[245]。

资质的保持

由于卒中治疗的领域日新月异，医生应该每两年接受至少16小时的卒中教育。此外，鼓励医生参与质量和改进监督项目。这个项目将审查卒中的急诊介入治疗质量和随访相关治疗效果[245,246]。

培训卒中救治团队

LVO卒中治疗的预后是时间依赖性的，已证明4.5小时时间窗外IVT的疗效会降低[75]。MT治疗的预后也同样显示了时间依赖性[188]。LVO卒中标准治疗方法是IVT联合MT来为患者带来更好的预后[248]。但是这需要组建多学科卒中团队来实现。为了最大限度地减少治疗时间和非技术性错误，建议应将仿真团队培训作为任何TSC的核心组成部分[249]。仿真的干预措施已被证明可以将入院到穿刺的时间间隔缩短12分钟，并可增加到院后30分钟内接受IVT的患者数量[250]。

3. 在您的社区建立取栓系统

许多高质量的临床试验表明，MT治疗AIS-LVO的患者具有显著的临床获益[10,14-16,18]。

重要的是，这些试验是在高容量的卒中中心开展的，并且这些中心拥有经验丰富的卒中专家，从而有能力为患者提供复杂的治疗。医疗机构的卒中救治团队由急诊科医生、放射科医生、神经介入医生、神经科医生、神经外科医生以及卒中培训的辅助人员组成。这些关键成员对于TSC提供高效的治疗至关重要[10,14-16,18,251]。

2016年，SVIN提出了促进LVO卒中系统发展的建议，包括将MT作为一种治疗方式[251]。这些建议补充了对目前综合性卒中中心的资格要求，包括高患者容量、先进的影像能力、院后协调治疗、专门的神经重症监护病房、质量控制、参与卒中研究和汇报绩效指标等。SVIN建议对这些标准进行如下补充。

- **高患者容量**

高容量的治疗措施与患者的良好预后息息相关[252-255]。建议需要每年应用MT治疗25~30例患者，TSC的所有神经介入医生应每年至少完成10次MT[251]。

- **先进的影像能力**

建议所有的TSC都具备能够治疗两名同时发生LVO卒中患者的能力；因此需要神经介入专家和相关的辅助人员随叫随到，卒中介入手术室随时可用[251]。

- **院后协调治疗**

推荐在TSC和康复中心之间建立监测和协调的系统，以确保后续的治疗。此类卒中后的治疗机构应获得卒中康复认证，工作人员应接受标准化的预后量表的培训[251]。

- **专门的神经重症监护病房**

由于AIS患者治疗管理的复杂性和潜在的并发症，由血管神经科医生和神经重症专家组成的多学科团队应随叫随到[251]。

- **同行评审过程**

建议目前建立的同行评审应纳入MT治疗与LVO卒中患者快速高效相关的绩效指标[251]。

- **参与卒中研究**

为提高质量，数据管理协调员应在所有TSC的工作人员中维护登记表，同时为分析提供临床数据[251]。

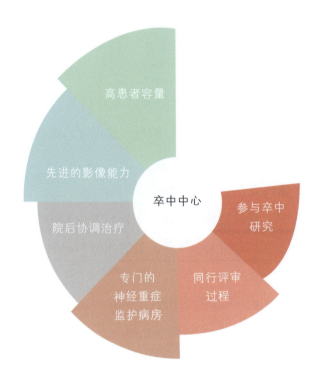

4. 改善 MT 的院间转诊

许多里程碑式临床试验有助于改进患者入院后的诊治流程系统,但入院前时间管理和根据患者症状严重程度分诊仍然是优化患者运输绩效指标的最重要因素[256]。越长入院-出院(DIDO)时间会对 LVO 卒中患者的预后产生不利的影响,这可能是发病-MT 治疗时间中最大的可控因素[257]。

院间转运的优点和缺点

多项里程碑式的试验已经证明 MT 能使患者获益[10,14-16,18]。因此,AHA/ASA 更新了 2013 年的指南,以反映改善卒中治疗系统的必要性,包括院前分诊、院间转诊和 TSC 认证[261]。将患者转运至 TSC 来让其接受MT。然而,MT 前的转院会延误诊治,并对 LVO 卒中患者的预后产生不利的影响[262]。早期识别LVO卒中后,直接将患者送至具备MT能力的TSC可获得更好的预后[264,265];因此EMS应直接将患者送至TSC而不是送至附近医院。为缩短转运时间,所有TSC都应具备MT的能力[266]。

无效转院原因

在2009—2014年,AIS的转院率增加了33%,MT的需求量加大[267]。法国的一项研究表明,45%的因MT而转院是无效的患者最终未能接受介入治疗,可能是因为转院期间血管闭塞增加导致临床症状恶化[268]。

影响MT延误的因素包括:最早发现人的识别、EMS的效率、院间转诊、通知MT团队以及流程内的延误[270]。侧支代偿情况、较高的NIHSS评分和初级转诊中心的CTA能独立预测转院后患者接受MT的概率[43]。

转院过程中的延误以及如何避免

DIDO时间是发病到再通时间最大的可校正因素,DIDO时间越长,对LVO卒中患者的预后越不利[257]。建立重症监护复苏中心可能会缩短转院时间,并有利于改善LVO卒中患者的预后[221]。

医院治疗流程的质量改进

通过质量改进可改善较远的TSC的MT延误[272]。许多临床试验有助于改善患者直接入院后的院内工作流程;但正如区域卒中管理系统的真实数据所显示的,院前时间管理和分诊仍然是优化患者转运的绩效指标的最重要因素。优化院内治疗流程对于预防转院的延误和MT的相关延误至关重要[49]。2017年SVIN的一篇报道建议,由于LVO卒中患者发病和死亡的风险不断攀升,需尽快实现再灌注,这取决于优化医院的诊治流程[50]。标准化TSC方案的一些特性包括尽早通知TSC、云数据共享和到院时的CTA,这与改善LVO卒中患者的预后相关[51,273]。详细的分层系统可以帮助减少不恰当的转运并改善预后[53]。

移动诊疗模式

卒中治疗的移动诊疗模式，是由可移动的卒中介入小组在 TSC 提供介入治疗，这比患者在最近的医院行 IVT 的逐级转运模式快了 79 分钟。因此，这种模式是在城市中院间转诊的一种潜在替代方案[274]。

卒中会诊选项

远程卒中会诊是一种专门从事卒中诊疗的专家通过技术手段帮助其他地区的卒中患者进行治疗，这种方案提高了卒中患者的 MT 治疗率，减少了转院的必要性[274]。

直升机紧急医疗服务

直升机紧急医疗服务（HEMS）的作用需要进一步明确，以便在转运过程中提供更好的辅助治疗，并消除患者由于地理位置的接受 MT 的差异[275]。

给政策制定者的建议

1. 给政策制定者的关键建议

（1）高容量卒中病例医院的医生和管理者。

（2）评估本地区的卒中和 LVO 的疾病负担。

（3）评估现有系统对于卒中管理的有效性，发现关键的缺陷。

（4）评估本地区现有系统的成本和疗效，并对您所在地区患者的临床和成本效益进行详细分析。

（5）制定一项旨在减轻卒中疾病负担和改善临床预后的政策。

（6）为可能从 MT 获益但经济能力有限的 LVO 患者建立基金。

（7）成立卒中教育项目，重点科普卒中症状、如何获得急救和可及的卒中系统资源。

（8）设立能够开展 MT 的区域性卒中中心。

（9）增加神经介入医生的培训数量，目标是获得足够的技能来治疗 LVO。

2. 患者诊疗路径的推荐步骤

临床病史

伊丽莎白，62岁女性，有心房颤动病史，口服华法林。晨起散步时突发左侧肢体无力。路过目击者呼叫 EMS，救护车 15 分钟内到达，识别了卒中的体征，将患者送至可行 MT 的卒中中心。

院内评估

到达卒中中心后，患者症状缓解，行头颅 CT 检查，未显示早期梗死或出血。

治疗

她接受了 IVT 治疗，到院到治疗时间为 45 分钟，发病到治疗时间为 90 分钟。CTA 提示大脑中动脉（MCA）闭塞，行 MT 治疗，采用取栓支架和动脉溶栓。术后影像未显示梗死负担。

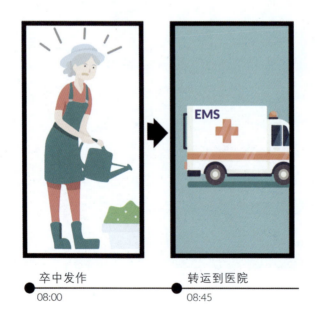

给政策制定者的建议

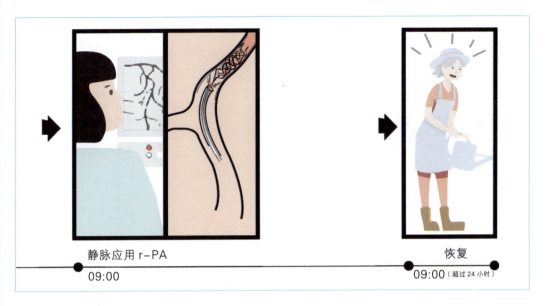

静脉应用 r-PA　　　　　恢复
09:00　　　　　　　　09:00（超过24小时）

结局

该患者临床预后很好，功能完全独立，第二天出院。

下一步

1. 和 SVIN 的成员讨论本报告，了解 MT 如何惠及您所在的区域。

2. 和主要利益相关方及决策者内部讨论医疗系统的卒中管理。

3. 组织临床专家及政策决策者开会来评价改进本地 LVO 治疗的必要性。

关于作者

SVIN：血管与介入神经病学学会

本报告由 SVIN 主要的血管和神经介入学专家撰写，代表了介入放射学的先进水平，目标是改善卒中和脑血管病患者的临床诊疗和预后。2016年，SVIN 发起了"取栓使命 2020"（Mission Thrombectomy 2020），初心是联合全球的力量改善卒中诊疗，截至 2020 年将年取栓例数从 100 000 例增加到 202 000 例，在全球范围内降低了卒中相关致疾率，挽救了成千上万人的生命。为了实施这个项目，SVIN 和政府组织、非盈利医疗机构以及行业领军人合作，提高公众意识，建立财务计划支持高级卒中中心的发展。

附 录

A. 机械取栓治疗急性卒中的文献综述和具体科学证据

1. 什么是卒中?

根据美国卒中学会（ASA）的定义，当大脑的血管被血栓堵塞或破裂导致局部脑组织缺氧和缺乏营养时，就会造成卒中。当大脑的供血动脉突然阻塞，导致脑血流速度迅速减慢或骤然停止时，就会造成急性缺血性卒中（AIS）的发生[34]。堵塞通常是由于脂肪沉积导致血管狭窄而形成血栓，或是身体其他部位的血栓进入并滞留在脑血管中所造成的。即便是几分钟的缺氧也可能造成永久性脑损伤[34]。缺氧环境会迅速杀死脑细胞，并导致明显的身体症状，如身体一侧突然出现面部、手臂或腿的麻木或无力，意识不清，视物困难，行走障碍或严重的头痛。更为罕见的非传统症状包括身体一侧出现面部、手臂或腿的疼痛，头晕，精神状态或意识的改变，头痛，一般神经系统症状（恶心、打嗝、非局灶性无力）和非神经系统症状（胸痛、心悸、气短）[41,35]等。

研究表明，女性更容易表现出非传统性卒中症状[35]，这导致女性患者中接受静脉溶栓治疗的比例要比男性低30%[36]。另有一些研究报道，女性卒中患者在院外和院内治疗上延误更久[37-46]。此外，卒中曾被视为是一种老年疾病，因为多数患者的发病年龄在65岁以上[29,30]，且在55岁之后，年龄每增长10岁，发病率会翻倍[47,48]。然而，中青年人群的卒中患病率随着肥胖者和糖尿病患者的增多正在逐年攀升[49]。

由此可见，随着世界人口的增多及人口老龄化，卒中患病率将继续增长[50,51]。

2. 在AIS中什么是LVO？

大血管闭塞（LVO）是指位于头和颈部的四根主要动脉之一的堵塞[52-59]。尽管LVO约占AIS全部发病人数的1/3，但与其他卒中亚型相比，其所致的卒中后3个月的残疾或死亡率显著更高[58,60,61]，这是因为LVO者梗死体积更大[62,63]，神经功能缺陷更为严重[64,65]。

LVO可以通过四种机制发生：继发于颅内动脉的动脉粥样硬化闭塞，颅外动脉粥样硬化性栓塞或斑块破裂导致颅内血管闭塞，与房颤等心脏疾病相关的心脏栓塞事件导致颅内血管闭塞，以及其他不明原因所致的血管闭塞[66]。LVO通常会导致供给脑组织的血流不足，进而造成细胞受损和炎症，最终导致神经元、神经胶质细胞和内皮细胞死亡[60]。尽管缺血性变化在数分钟之内就会发生，但最终的梗死体积取决于低灌注的程度和时间[67]；流向缺血区的侧支循环水平在卒中进展中起很大作用。

3. 有哪些治疗方式可供选择？

对可疑AIS的患者，在根据神经影像的结果排除颅内出血后，可考虑使用药物溶栓和血管内治疗，并给予一般支持治疗。在治疗过程中预测和监测急性医源性并发症或卒中相关的神经系统并发症。最后，评估本次卒中最可能的病因，并围绕对缺血性事件复发的预防展开治疗。

可根据卒中中心的能力选择以下任何一种治疗方式。

用溶栓药物（静脉 t-PA）进行静脉溶栓

静脉溶栓（IVT）/使用溶栓药物（阿替普酶，又名组织型纤溶酶原激活物，t-PA）是唯一被 FDA 批准用于治疗 AIS 的药物，使用后可改善患者预后。尽管一些研究表明遗传差异、种族和性别可能会影响 t-PA 的疗效，但研究也发现只有某些共患病，如高血压（血压升高）和高血糖（血糖升高），才会给 AIS 患者的溶栓反应带来显著的负面影响[70-74]。

机械取栓

MT 用于解除 LVO，逆转神经功能缺损。MT 的操作过程：

- 将导管置入股动脉内，并上送通过颈部血管，抵达造成卒中的血栓处。
- 在 X 线影像引导下，将回收支架经导管置入微导管内。
- 支架穿过血栓，释放支架并撑开已闭塞的动脉使血液流通，然后被"回收"（或者叫回撤），从而移除血栓。

静脉 t-PA 溶栓联合 MT

在卒中发病 4.5 小时内采取静脉 t-PA 溶栓能显著提高 AIS 患者中良好预后的比例，且这一效应不受年龄或卒中严重程度的影响，但颅内出血的风险也会随之增加。因此，如无禁忌，IVT 是所有发病 4.5 小时内的 AIS 患者的标准治疗方法[75]。然而，IVT 有一些重要的局限性，例如治疗时间窗很短，这就导致随着时间延长溶栓疗效迅速下降，且很多患者会超窗而无法得到治疗[75]。其他缺陷还包括溶栓组与安慰剂组相比，其总体致命性脑出血发生率增加[75]，血栓负担量大的患者再通率很低[76]，以及各种溶栓禁忌证限制了其应用，例如溶栓前服用过口服抗凝剂和症状

急性卒中机械取栓：现状与经验

出现时间不明者。

仅为 4.5 小时的狭窄时间窗和众多的禁忌证使得许多患者无法接受治疗——只有不到 3% 的 AIS 患者能接受静脉注射 rt-PA[9]。静脉溶栓联合机械取栓有可能会克服单纯 IVT 的局限性，尤其是对 LVO 再通率低的问题[75]。

自 2014 年 10 月起，8 项应用了新型器械的随机对照试验的结果一致表明，相比单纯药物治疗，MT 结合药物治疗可显著改善前循环大血管闭塞所致的缺血性卒中患者的预后[10]。

4. 机械取栓：新的治疗标准

卒中的起病急、疗效呈时间依赖的特性导致其治疗具有很大难度。对于未接受治疗的卒中而言，每分钟可破坏 200 万个神经元、140 亿个突触和累计 12 千米的有髓纤维。总的来说，这些神经变化每发生 1 小时，相当于大脑老化 3.6 年，这就使得患者尽快接受治疗显得至关重要[6]。

有效溶栓的时间窗很短，因为大多数患者必须在 4.5 小时内进行治疗[77]，且患者的预后取决于症状出现到再通之间的时间间隔，以及再通成功与否[78,79]。大量随机试验表明，与溶栓相比，MT 加快了再通，改善了患者的预后，并延长了治疗时间窗[9,11,12,15,16,18,26,32]。

MT 是一种微创手术，其使用微导管和其他取栓器械来机械性抓取和清除闭塞动脉中的血凝块。

根据其作用机制，MT 器械可分为不同的亚型：①线圈型取栓器；②抽吸装置；③可回收支架；④使用激光或超声波的机械性血块崩解器。

目前应用最多的是取栓支架和抽吸装置。取栓支架是由一根可扩张的管状金属网制成的，目的是将血栓完整地取出。取栓支架经输送导管置入，一旦放置到位，金属网释放将血栓捕获，然后整体收入导管内并从患者体内取出[80]。

抽吸导管内径更大，更灵活。将导丝置入患者体内后，沿其置入小导引导管用于引导抽吸导管到位。抵达血栓部位后，血栓将被分解成小碎片后经抽吸导管用泵吸或手动将血栓碎片吸出[154]。

在最近的研究中，由采用大口径导管的抽吸取栓联合可回收支架的机械性取栓疗法展现出了良好的前景[81]。在这项技术中，首先尝试使用大口径抽吸导管抽吸血栓（因这种选择更便宜）。如果抽吸失败，则通过抽吸导管插入可回收支架来进行机械取栓。这种有序组合使血管再通率高达95%[81]，而仅直接抽吸取栓的再通率为78%。

5. 卒中与 LVO 的发生率：全球视角

卒中的人口学特征

卒中目前是全球第二大死因和主要致残原因之一[51,82]。2016年，全球缺血性卒中患病数为6760万，出血性卒中患病数为1530万[83]。东欧、中亚和东亚国家的缺血性卒中患病率最高[83]。2010年，全球约发生了1160万次缺血性卒中；在该年中，63%的缺血性卒中和80%的出血性卒中发生在低收入国家和中等收入国家[84]。

2016年，全球有550万人死于脑血管病。1990—2016年，在死亡人数增加28.2%的同时，年龄标准化死亡率却下降了36.2%[84]；最近的一份报告表明，美国近年来卒中死亡率的下降趋势并未持续[85]。东欧和中东亚国家的缺血性卒中死亡率最高[84]。2010年，估计有3940万个残疾调整寿命年（DALY）因缺血性卒中而损失[84]。同年，高收入国家与卒中相关的死亡平均年龄为80.4岁，而低收入和中等收入国家为72.1岁[86]。

卒中与几个可控和不可控的危险因素有关。年龄、性别、人种和民族是卒中的不可控危险因素，而高血压、高脂血症、房颤、吸烟、肥胖、糖尿病、颈动脉或其他动脉疾病、饮食、缺乏体力活动、腰臀比、心理社会

急性卒中机械取栓：现状与经验

因素、心脏原因和饮酒被认为是可改变的危险因素[87-91]。在全球范围内，这些因素占卒中可控风险的近90%[88]。据估计，50%的卒中是可以通过控制前五个最相关的可控危险因素（高血压、高脂血症、房颤、吸烟及肥胖）来预防的[92]，因此，国际社会在该领域的专家已经把预防卒中列为优先事项[93]。

在可控的卒中危险因素中，高血压是发达国家和发展中国家普遍存在的[94]，而且是卒中的唯一最重要的危险因素。在最近的一项荟萃分析中，有9项研究表明血压控制在<150/90 mmHg可减少卒中，6项研究表明，较低的血压控制范围（≤140/85 mmHg）与卒中的显著降低相关[95-97]。另一项临床研究的荟萃分析表明，抗高血压治疗收缩压降低10 mmHg或舒张压降低5mmHg，可使卒中发病率平均下降41%[98]，最近的一份特别报告指出了高血压治疗在全球范围内降低卒中风险的积极意义[99]。

根据一项多国家的荟萃分析结果，糖尿病是卒中的独立危险因素，1/3的卒中患者患有糖尿病[100]。糖尿病对女性的影响比男性更为突出[101,102]。此外，患有糖尿病的成年人罹患卒中的风险高出两倍[103]，卒中占这类人群死亡原因的20%[104,105]。而随着糖尿病病程的延长，卒中的风险也在逐渐增加[104]。缺血性卒中的糖尿病患病率为33%[100]。有趣的是，糖尿病缺血性卒中患者往往更年轻（非裔美国人在55岁之前，白人在65岁之前）；与非糖尿病患者相比，非裔美国人更有可能患有至少一种合并症，如高血压、高脂血症和心肌梗死[106]。

卒中过去被认为是一种老龄化人口的疾病，大多数卒中发生在65岁以上的人群中[29,30]，发病率在55岁后每10年会翻番[47,48]。在美国，35~44岁的成年人卒中的发病率为每年30~120/10万，65~74岁的成年人每年为670~970/10万[107,108]。与年轻的卒中患者相比，年龄正常也与死亡率的升高以及生活质量下降相关[109-114]。然而，在过去的几十年中，全世界年龄<65岁的人群卒中发生率增加了25%[115]，尤其是在低收入

和中等收入国家，例如俄罗斯、中国和印度。这种卒中负担的转移考虑与年轻人群心血管疾病风险不断上升相关[51,116-121]。性别也被认为会影响卒中的发病与预后。总体来说，女性有着更高的卒中患病率，因为女性的预期寿命长于男性；然而男性在其生命的大多数时间里卒中的发病风险更高，这些数据趋势并非特定于某个地理区域[36,96,122-125]）。

根据2016年全球疾病负担（GBD）研究卒中患者终身风险显示，据估计，2016年全球25岁及以上人群卒中的终身风险接近25%，男性和女性的发病率几乎相等[126]。缺血性卒中的风险高于出血性卒中的风险。此外，研究发现卒中的终身风险根据社会-人口统计指数（SDI）和GBD区域的不同而有所改变。最高和最低的卒中风险分别与中高SDI和低SDI相关；然而，研究也发现低卒中风险可能是由于多种死亡原因的发生率较高，而并不一定是卒中风险的真正降低[49,126,127]。全球各地区的数据比较显示，东亚、中欧和东欧的卒中终身风险最高，撒哈拉以南非洲的终身风险最低[126]。这些数据是根据卒中的发生率以及卒中以外其他原因导致死亡的风险来估计的。总体来说，低SDI国家例如撒哈拉沙漠以南非洲是由于其他原因致死风险较高而导致更低的终身卒中风险，因此，风险的降低并不一定表示这些国家的卒中发生率更低[126]。

6. LVO的发病率——人口学统计

在美国，LVO的发病率估计在每年24/100 000[47,56]，同时每年大概有80万例AIS发生[3,47]。在美国，大约有8万例AIS是由于LVO导致的[47]。大约一半的卒中相关死亡与AIS相关[5]。在所有AIS的病例中，已有11%~46%的病例报告称是由于LVO引起的[47,53,55,114-116]。颅内大血管闭塞如颈内动脉（ICA）末端、大脑中动脉（MCA）和基底动脉（BA），被认为是严重的并且与高死亡率与发病率有关。

急性卒中机械取栓:现状与经验

根据 Lakomkin 等人对 AIS 患者 LVO 的患病率进行的 10 年系统性回顾(2019 年),尽管受限于不同医疗机构之间定义和报告方法上的差异,其预估的准确性、AIS 患者 LVO 的患病率要高于预期[87]。在已有的研究中,AIS 患者 LVO 的患病率在 7.3%~60.6%。在 17 组患者中(Vanacker 等人描述的 AIS 患者队列的推导和验证)[57],LVO 的发生率平均为 31.1%,当根据每项研究中包含的患者数量进行加权后,平均发病率为 29.3%[87]。

美国

在美国,卒中的年发病率约为 80 万,是全国第五大死因,每年导致超过 14.6 万人死亡(每 19 人中有 1 人死亡),并且也是导致严重残疾的主要原因,这使许多人长期残疾并且无法工作[117]。在美国,卒中的患病率在 20 岁或 20 岁以上的人群中为 2.7%(共计 720 万人),并且随着年龄的增长而增加。60 岁以上和 80 岁以上人群的患病率分别为 6% 和 13%[117]。考虑到所有卒中类型,AIS 几乎占到了 87%[43]。

由于 LVO 导致的 AIS,包括大脑中动脉、颈内动脉末端和基底动脉,年发病率估计大概在每年 24/10 万人,相当于每年接近 8 万例 LVO 病例[47]。最近几项随机对照试验研究了前循环 LVO 的患者(包括 ICA)[10,14,15,26],平均年龄在 65~70 岁,其患病率在年龄上没有明显差异。将这些研究放在一起分析,发现吸烟、糖尿病、房颤和高血压与 LVO 显著相关[10,14,15,26]。

中国

在中国,卒中是首要的致死原因,占到了 22.45%,其中 65% 都是 AIS[118]。此外,35%~40% 的 AIS 是由于近端大血管动脉粥样硬化性狭窄或闭塞导致的[116]。最近的一项针对中国主要急诊医疗机构 6809 名 AIS 患者的研究显示,AIS 患者相比非 LVO 患者的年龄更大(平均年龄为 80.5 岁 vs 71.4 岁),拥有更高的 30 天死亡率(31.1% vs 4.6%)以及更长的平均住院日（平均 38.6 天 *vs* 21.1 天）[119]。

日本

2017 年，卒中是日本第三大死亡原因[120]，在经过年龄和性别校正后，卒中发病率为每年 142.9/10 万人（采用 2013 年欧洲标准人群确定；95%CI 123.3~168.5）。缺血性卒中的发病率为每年 91.3/10 万人[121]。

中东地区：沙特阿拉伯

中东地区社会、经济和环境条件的转变导致生活方式的急剧变化，同时也导致了卒中负担的增高[122]。最近的一项系统综述囊括了 1980—2015 年 5 月中东地区卒中相关的文献[122]。卒中的发病率为每年 22.7~250/10 万人，患病率为 508~777/10 万人。卒中在男性中比在女性中更为常见，并且平均发病年龄在 60~80 岁。缺血性卒中是最常见的卒中类型，而高血压和糖尿病是最常见的卒中相关危险因素[122]。

沙特阿拉伯的卒中患病率估计在 0.67%[123]。1998 年报告的首次卒中的发病率为每年 29.8/10 万人[124]；然而，考虑到目前的人口数量，发病率预估已经增加到每年 50.9/10 万人[125]。最近的一项研究调查了沙特阿拉伯西南部 Aseer 地区的卒中发病率，研究纳入了 2016 年 1 月 1 日到 2016 年 12 月 31 日期间入住 Aseer 医院的 1249 名首次卒中的患者[126]。根据患者的人口学统计，发病率为每年 57.64/10 万人，这与预计的数据相符；但是，发病率随着年龄的增长在逐渐增加，在 70 岁以上的人群中发病率达到了每年 851.81/10 万人。研究发现，卒中在男性中更为常见[126]。沙特阿拉伯的卒中患者治疗标准低于其他发达国家，这导致接近 95% 的患者并没有在专业的卒中中心接受治疗；而无论卒中的类型，即使是 LVO，也仅仅接受了非再灌注治疗[127]。

印度

印度的人口、经济和流行病学发生了重大变化[128]，这导致了预期寿命的延长和老龄化人口的增加[129,130]。这进一步导致了印度高收入地区卒中发生率下降了42%（从1970—1979年的每年163/10万人下降到2000—2008年的每年94/10万人）[131]。2014年的一项回顾性研究分析了印度高级医疗中心进行血管内治疗的AIS-LVO患者的预后[132,149]。所有患者均有溶栓禁忌证或者在进行血管内治疗前静脉溶栓失败。45例患者被纳入研究，患者平均年龄为49±14岁，71%（32/45）的患者是男性。在90天后的随访中，64%的患者拥有良好预后，同时36%的患者预后较差，包括18%的患者死亡[132]。

丹麦

最近的一项回顾性研究分析了2011—2017年丹麦卒中登记的所有急性血管内再灌注治疗AIS-LVO患者的数据[133]。被纳入的1720例患者的中位年龄为70岁，其中58%为男性。卒中-LVO患者从2011年的128例明显增加到2017年的409例。发病3个月时，45%的患者预后良好，43%的患者预后不良。总体而言，1年死亡率为22%，生存率从2011年的96例大幅增加到2016年的994例[133]。

7. LVO治疗的差距

大量的研究和临床试验证实了溶栓治疗在一个特定的治疗窗口内对改善AIS患者的临床预后和康复的有效性。AIS患者的首要治疗目标是及时恢复尚未梗死的可挽救的缺血脑组织的血流[155]。使血栓溶解的再灌注治疗[156]，包括静脉t-PA和血管内干预如MT，是唯一被批准的治疗AIS的治疗方法。当作为单一疗法使用时，这两种治疗方法都有局限性。唯一批准用于治疗

AIS 的药物是静脉 rt-PA（重组 t-PA）；然而，它对 LVO 导致的 AIS 患者无效，这是因为其血栓负荷量大。这限制了 LVO 治疗的选择。

在这类患者中，MT 被证明更有效。目前，再灌注患者选择的主要标准是卒中症状出现的时间。静脉 t-PA 必须在症状出现后 4.5 小时的时间窗内进行再灌注治疗，MT 则必须在 6~8 小时内进行再灌注治疗。静脉 t-PA 治疗的限制是时间超过 4.5 小时，这使得超过该时间窗的大多数卒中患者丧失了溶栓治疗的资格[157-160]（约 85%），因此大大限制了符合条件的人群[157-160]。

静脉 rt-PA 的其他限制包括：

（1）增加了颈内动脉闭塞（ICA）[156,161-163] 或其他致残卒中（如没有检测到残余血流信号的卒中）的死亡率和颅内出血的概率[164-166]。

（2）对 LVO 的再通率低（13%~50%），如近端大脑中动脉（MCA）、ICA 或基底动脉[167]。

（3）对长段血栓无作用（特别是当血栓长度超过 8mm 或位于近端时，如颈动脉终末闭塞[165]。

一项研究发现只有 10% 和 25% 的 ICA 和近端 MCA 闭塞可通过静脉 rt-PA 再通[168]。在静脉 rt-PA 治疗的患者中经常观察到不完全再通。例如，70% 接受静脉 rt-PA 治疗的患者被发现有血管造影证实的残余血栓，需要行血管内治疗，如血管成形术[169]。

除了以上的局限，静脉 rt-PA 在 AIS 中的应用还有几个禁忌证[167]。

这些局限和禁忌极大地限制了对卒中患者的治疗选择，尤其是大多数 LVO 患者。考虑到静脉 rt-PA 的限制导致其只在不到 3% 的卒中患者中使用，卒中治疗的拓展不应在溶栓药物上，而应是在血管内介入治疗如 MT 上。

8. 神经介入医生的短缺

神经介入学是神经放射学的一个分支，它可以通过将血管内的各种器

急性卒中机械取栓：现状与经验

械推送至先前确定的病变部位来实现微创治疗。据估计，在美国每年进行取栓手术率为3/10万，每年的取栓例数为1万例[46,57]。因此，手术例数大大低于LVO的发生率，这表明取栓手术例数和使用率在未来还有很大的提升空间。

世界卫生组织统计，每年有500万人死于卒中[134]。随着人口老龄化的增长，这些数字预计还会增加。LVO卒中的发病率增高预计将增加对神经取栓手术器械、神经介入医生、取栓手术和有能力开展取栓手术的医院的需求[135]。

目前，美国有超过200家综合卒中中心[136]。美国卒中治疗市场正在迅速增长，这主要得益于AIS器械市场的扩张，预计到2026年，这个市场规模将翻番[136]。美国卒中治疗模式正在向专业的高容量卒中治疗中心转移，并将患者直接运送到这些有取栓能力的综合中心，以便更及时地开始治疗。但综合卒中中心认证过程既费时又费钱，这限制了这些中心的发展；而且农村/人口稀少的地区人群继续得不到及时的治疗，因为在该地区，建立新医院是不合理的。但是，由于AIS器械和取栓手术费用在美国是全部报销的，预计卒中治疗的数量将在未来10年大幅增加。

2012年，Zaidat等人的一项研究估计了每年满足MT标准的AIS患者数量和训练有素的神经介入医生的需求量[137]。据估计，在以大城市为中心的50英里范围内，约有800名神经介入医生执业，覆盖了美国95%以上的人口。每年大约有40名神经介入医生从美国培训项目中毕业。这项研究开始10年后，神经介入医生的人数估计为1200人。每位神经介入医生每年估计完成22~81例MT。该研究得出的结论是，即使需要MT的AIS病例数量增加，目前和预计的神经介入医生数量也足以满足未来的需求。

这一发现已得到该领域其他专家的证实。David Fiorella和Harry Cloft在回应Zaidat文章的信中声称，新毕业生将继续在已经被神经介入服务覆盖的人口过剩地区出现[138]。过度增长的神经介入医生数量分散了卓越中心的护理和减少了容量,因此,随着每位神经介入医生的容量减少,护理可能会恶化。容积标准面积是由专业社会推荐的,因为患者的结果表明,增加病例量和操作经验可能会更好[139]。

然而,神经介入医生数量过多也受到了其他研究的质疑。Avasarala 和 Wesley 根据一项观察性电子邮件调查的结果,讨论了神经介入医生在不断变化的卒中治疗系统中所承担的责任[140]。神经内科医生必须在卒中患者到达后 15 分钟内赶到患者床边。此外,基于主观调查的数据,医生的职业倦怠正在升级,一些研究称之为危机[141]。研究估计,到 2025 年,神经内科医生的人才缺口将达到 19%[142]。

欧洲

在整个欧洲,各国对神经介入医生的需求有很大差异。像德国这样的国家有足够数量的能够提供 MT 的神经介入医生,而其他国家则没有。瑞士伯尔尼大学在 2017 年欧洲微侵袭神经治疗学会(ESMINT)年会(法国尼斯)上的报告估计,基于以下研究,仅有 20% 的欧洲患者能够接受 MT。

来自瑞士的一项研究表明,在症状出现 6 小时内到综合卒中中心就诊的卒中患者中,10.5% 符合基于 AHA/ASA 指南的 MT 的适应证[143]。

在格拉斯哥,真实数据显示,大约 15% 的发病 6 小时内的患者可能符合 MT 的适应证[144]。研究发现,临床试验的入组标准要严格得多;这项研究中大约 1% 的患者符合最近所有试验的入组标准。一项来自瑞典医院的研究估计了未来对取栓手术的需求。2016 年,欧洲专业组织发布了新的治疗指南[145]。与之前的指南相比,MT 的适应证不是那么严格了。作者估计,如果该指南在 2013 年发布,MT 的数量将会提高 5 倍[146]。

因此,在欧洲 130 万急性卒中患者中,估计每年有 13 万~23 万患者可能需要血管内治疗[147]。

急性卒中机械取栓：现状与经验

非洲

非洲卒中治疗的系统综述强调了现有的数据有限，并明确了非洲卒中治疗的差距，不同国家中和环境下，卒中治疗的频率远低于推荐标准[148,184]。只有14/54（25.9%）的非洲国家有相关文献报告。在医疗运输、CT/MRI成像技术、卒中病房、药物/溶栓、康复服务和医疗保健人员等方面都有短缺。Urimubenshi等人总结说，非洲的政策制定者和医疗专家需要共同努力，改善卒中治疗，确保尽可能多的患者获得治疗。

中东

Al-Senani等人在2019年发表的一项沙特阿拉伯的最新研究发现，目前可用的工作人员和卒中治疗服务不足以跟上预计增加的卒中病例，特别是在急症和康复服务领域[185]。作者认为，为了满足这些需求，需要对现有员工和服务进行重组，并在多个领域对新员工进行大量投资。10年间增编工作人员的费用总额估计约为2.3亿美元。

亚洲

在日本，卒中专家的数量与美国相似。可达性因地区而异，人口少的农村地区的可达性最低[150]。高达17.5%的老年人住在距离治疗机构60分钟路程或更远的地方[186]。此外，卒中专家的分布与医院的床位和医生的数量也不匹配。

9. MT实施协议

卒中治疗系统允许协调和整合整个卒中治疗的连续流程，包括社区教育、预防、紧急医疗服务、配备卒中治疗单元的综合卒中中心、介入专家、溶栓和MT，以及协调康复医院和服务。在全球范围内，增加高度发达的卒中系统每年能挽救近200万人的生命[28]，这主要取决于多少患者进入该卒中系统的情况[187]。由于血管疾病的老龄化和迅速增长的发生率，增加患者到综合卒中系统治疗的概率是10年内主要的紧迫公共卫生焦点之一。

在AIS-LVO的患者中，MT联合溶栓治疗使神经系统[改良Rankin评分（mRS）0~2]预后良好的概率增加了一倍以上[188]。在一项对五项主要临床试验的荟萃分析中评估了MT与单纯溶栓治疗相比的安全性和有效性，46%接受MT治疗的患者在90天时的mRS为0~2，而在接受单纯溶栓治疗的患者中只有26.5%[188]。此外，26.9%接受MT治疗的患者能达到主要的神经功能恢复（mRS 0~1），而只接受溶栓治疗的患者只有12.9%[188]。另外，在一项旨在确定MT与单独溶栓相比的安全性和有效性的前瞻性观察性研究中，发现90.4%（458/504）单独接受MT治疗的患者，92.4%（557/603）接受MT联合溶栓治疗的患者实现部分或完全血管再通[189]。这与仅溶栓治疗相比，是一个巨大的进步，因为单纯接受溶栓治疗的患者中只有60.0%（926/1543）实现了明显的血管再通[189]。实际上，与单纯溶栓相比每100名接受MT治疗的患者中，有38名患者遗留更少的卒中相关残疾，而58名将实现神经功能恢复和功能独立性[188]。

卒中的治疗是一个复杂的、多步骤的过程，需要及时、有效的治疗，以增加良好预后的可能性。在建设有效的卒中治疗系统时，从患者的角度出发，体验是至关重要的。

10. MT的临床获益

MT被认为是卒中治疗的突破。从脑部清除血栓可为卒中患者带来更好的预后，包括更大的功能独立和自由活动的可能性。之前的血管介入治疗无法迅速、安全地清除血栓。

急性卒中机械取栓：现状与经验

在研究卒中发作后 6 小时内 MT 对 LVO 患者疗效的初步试验中，为了最大限度地增加可挽救性组织的数量并增加手术受益的概率，大面积梗死的患者被排除在外[14-16,18]。这种可挽救的脑组织称为半暗带，这是缺血组织周围存在的可能发展为梗死（组织死亡）的区域，但如果再灌注则可以避免发展为梗死。随后的临床试验使用了 CT 或磁共振灌注成像来辨别缺血半暗带。缺血半暗带是核心梗死区周围的有延迟或接近正常血流灌注的区域，因卒中导致显著的血流减少[9,26,87]。这些试验已经证明，MT 对某些症状发作后长达 24 小时的适当半暗带/核心比的 LVO 患者具有疗效[9,26,87]。

在过去的 20 年中，随着基于循证证据的卒中检测的发展、高级治疗的普及及对卒中应急管理的改进，卒中的治疗发生了翻天覆地的转变[88]。2015 年之前，卒中都是用溶栓药物 t-PA 治疗，这种治疗因只能在卒中发生后 4.5 小时的狭窄治疗窗内而使用受限，这使很多 AIS 患者无法进行溶栓治疗[89,90]。此后，随着血管内器械的研发，AIS 的治疗方法发生了巨大变化，将这种器械置入股动脉，沿血管到达颈部，直至到达血栓并捕获、移除它。尽管这些器械经历了几次演变，2015 年却是具有里程碑意义的一年——5 项随机试验证明，机械取栓在清除血栓和挽救脑功能方面比药物治疗有效得多，后来的研究也证实了这一点（MR CLEAN, EXTEND-IA, ESCAPE, SWIFT PRIME, REVASCAT, DAWN 和 DEFUSE）[9,10,14-18,26]。这些研究表明，MT 治疗 24 小时内的卒中发作有巨大益处，这给卒中治疗带来了革命性的变化：从单纯的药物治疗转变为介入治疗，从而使功能预后良好的患者人数平均增加了 21.4%[9,10,14-18,26]。

这些研究使 MT 得到了普及，在短短 3 年内，手术总数翻了一倍，并有望以每年 25% 的速度增长，到 2025 年将达到 103 000 例。2018 年美国卒中协会指南建议对 AIS 患者进行紧急取栓[87]。

11. MT 的经济效益

卒中治疗的有效性对时间敏感,卒中发病到治疗的时间越短,其预后转归率、再通率、再灌注率越高且死亡率越低[9,10,14-18,26]。良好的预后可降低经济负担。实际上,AIS(≤ 6 小时)患者及时得到治疗可缩短住院和康复周期,因此与较长时间才得到治疗(> 6 小时)的 AIS 患者相比,可降低成本[205]。与更长的治疗时间窗或不能再通相比,联合治疗(MT 联合静脉 t-PA)可提高卒中发作后 6 小时内的再通率,从而显著改善患者预后。

北美

美国

在美国,AIS 带来了很高的经济负担,特别是卒中相关残疾的出院患者;与非残疾患者相比,其费用要高出一倍以上($ 120 753 *vs* $ 54 580)[206]。虽然联合疗法(MT 联合静脉 t-PA)的住院初始费用($ 17 183)比标准疗法(溶栓药物)更高,但由于残疾率大幅下降,每位患者终身可节省 $ 23 203,并提高了整体生活质量。此外,联合疗法还可以降低卒中后的康复和护理(90 天的费用)以及终身费用,同时也使 QALY 增加了 1.74[20]。

2019 年,一项针对 11 800 名接受 MT 治疗的患者的研究发现,与标准治疗相比,接受 MT 治疗的患者的住院时间显著减少(8.7 天 *vs* 11.7 天),出院率增加(17.7% *vs* 29.6%)并且死亡率降低(21.6% *vs* 12.8%)[207]。总体而言,MT 可以降低 AIS 患者对公共和个人造成的经济负担。

2018 年的一项荟萃分析评估了联合治疗相对于患者年龄(50~100 岁)的成本效益[208]。研究发现,MT 对 50 岁患者的获益(2.61 分 QALY)和节省的费用最大(健康管理角度为 $ 99 555,社会角度为 $ 146 385)。

对于80岁的患者，联合治疗成功后，每增加一个质量调整生命年，增加的治疗效益（1.13 QALY）和成本（$19 041）与增加的1670美元的增量成本-效益比（ICER）有关。在$50 000/QALY为自愿支付门槛的情况下，MT的可接受率很高，为97.8%。尽管90岁患者的成本效益比增加到$35 802/QALY，当自愿支付门槛分别为$50 000/QALY，$100 000/QALY和$150 000/QALY时，可接受率仍然很高，分别为81.4%，99.1%和99.8%。因此，尽管手术费用很高，但对于79岁以下的患者，与单独进行标准治疗相比，联合卒中治疗可减少终身的直接和间接费用。而对于80~100岁的患者，他们可以体验到增加质量调整生命年的好处，而终身成本仅微幅增长[208]。

加拿大

加拿大AIS平均每年的花费成本为28亿美元，每位患者的平均成本为75 353美元/年[209]。与美国的数据相似，卒中相关残疾患者的年平均成本是非残疾患者的两倍以上（$107 883 vs $48 339）[209]。在5年的时间范围内，接受联合疗法的AIS-LVO患者的总费用略高于标准疗法（$126 939 vs $124 419），同时QALY升高（1.484 vs 1.273），相关ICER为$11 990/QALY。在自愿支付门槛为$50 000/QALY和$100 000/QALY的情况下，接受率高达89.7%和99.6%[210]，对AIS患者进行联合治疗预计可为加拿大医疗系统每年节省$321 334[211]。

欧洲

英国

在英国，联合治疗相比标准治疗，初始住院费用较高（$64 757.28 vs $52 494.73）；但是，QALY在6小时、12小时和24小时的增量成本分别为$1564（£1219），$5253（£4096）和$3712（£2894）；因此，这证明了这种治疗在卒中发作后24小时是有成本效益的，并且应该在英国国家医疗服务体系实行[212]。有趣的是，在英国，联合疗法在短期内（90天）是不划算的，但预计在20年后和终身范围具有一定的成本效益[213,214]。如果得以全面开展，则预计5年其价值可达到13亿英镑（17亿美元）[214]。

与标准治疗相比，联合疗法在每位患者身上的成本增加了12 262英镑，并且在20年里，每位患者的QALY增加了1.05，联合疗法的净货币收益也更高，每位患者总共节省了33 190英镑（43 437美元）[215]，表明MT对AIS患者具有成本效益[213]。

法国

与美国的结果相仿，在法国，联合治疗的初始住院费用比标准治疗高2116美元。然而，这些患者在卒中后90天的功能独立性增加了10.9%（53% vs 42.1%，$P = 0.028$）。对于每一个获得功能独立性的病例，ICER估值为19379美元，低于自愿支付门槛的36351美元（截至2015年），净货币收益为1853美元；因此，联合治疗带来的好处胜过手术本身的费用[216]。

卒中后1年，联合治疗患者的QALY得分高于标准治疗患者（0.58 vs 0.46）。预计每增加QALY所需的成本为14 880美元，并且预计的净货币收益为2757美元，即为MT一年的成本效益[216]。卒中后10年，成本效益仍保持在98%的高水平，并且每增加QALY，自愿支付门槛达到50 000欧元（55 797美元）[217]。

瑞典

在瑞典，MT手术会增加介入成本（$11 779），但由于对家庭医疗或疗养院护理的依赖较少（家庭帮助服务$17014，疗养院护理$34027），从长远来看会节省大量费用[218]。此外，联合治疗还可以提高生活质量（0.99 QALY）和预期寿命（0.40生命年），并且还会减少费用（$221）[219]。

意大利

从意大利国家医疗服务体系的角度来看，AIS-LVO 患者的联合治疗在卒中后的第 1 年和第 3 年之间具有成本效益，从第 4 年起可以节省费用。在第 1 年，MT 比标准治疗贵 € 4078.37（$4553.77）[€ 13 430.81（$14 996.37） vs € 9352.44（$10 442.61）]，QALY 为 0.17，ICER 为 € 23 990.44（$ 26 786.89）。在第 2 年和第 3 年，每位患者的总费用差异减小，而有效性的差异增大，ICER 为 € 6696（$7476.52）和 € 798（$891.02）。在第 5 年，与标准治疗相比，联合治疗的费用减少为 € 3057（$3411）[€ 31 798（$35 483） vs € 34 855（$38 895）]，并且 QALY 增为 0.77。因此，与标准治疗相比，AIS-LVO 患者的联合治疗具有更低的总费用和更好的预后[220]。

西班牙

从西班牙国家医疗服务体系的角度来看，与标准治疗相比，联合疗法的治疗费用较高 [€ 8428.00（$9405） vs € 1606.00（$1792）]，总体费用较低 [€ 123 866（$138 228） vs € 168 244（$187 752）]，以及净货币收益 € 119 744（$133 628）[自愿支付的门槛为 € 30 000（$33 478）/质量调整生命年][221]，研究结果与美国的结果相吻合。接受联合治疗患者的健康状况也得到了改善，延长了 1.17 个生命年和 2.51 分 QALY。因此，与单独的标准治疗相比，对 AIS-LVO 患者采用联合疗法成本更低且预后更好[221]。

澳大利亚

与美国的结果相吻合，联合治疗在澳大利亚具有更高的医院成本指数（每位患者 $10 666），生活质量更高；但与标准治疗相比，每位患者终身可节省超过 $8000 [222]。在最初的 90 天里，与标准治疗相比，接受联合治疗患者的平均住院费用更少（$15 689 vs $30 569，P = 0.008），抵消了医院间运输（平均 $573）和 MT 的额外费用（平均 $10 515）。平均每位患者可节省 $4365（$29 371 vs $33 736）。MT 治疗患者拥有更短的住院时间（5 天 vs 8 天）和康复时间（0 天 vs 27 天），健康寿命年数（DALYs）的损失降低了，生活质量提高了（9.3 vs 4.9 QALYs）。接受标准治疗患者的寿命延长了 4.4 年[11]。因此我们推测，使用联合治疗可减轻患者的经济负担。重要的是，与改良 Rankin 评分（mRS）相关的以患者为中心的评估（例如活动能力、自我护理、日常活动、疼痛/不适和焦虑/抑郁），对患者的预后影响最大[11]。

亚洲

中国

在中国，联合治疗在卒中后最初的 5 年内，并不具有成本效益，但在 6 年以后，则具有成本效益，并显著提高了优质生命年限。联合疗法的终生获益为 0.794 QALYs，额外费用为 50 030 元（7700 美元），每获得 QALY 的费用为 63 010 元（9690 美元）[223]。

结论

我们对 MT 的成本效益进行了全球分析。与标准治疗相比，MT 随着时间延长显示出了其效益。这可能与生存和生活质量的提高和长期治疗的减少（如护理和康复设备等）有关。AIS 的经济研究大多来自发达国家，但正扩展至新的区域，成本可能根据年龄、流程分型以及患者状态基线进行划分。

12. 实施MT的挑战

有可靠数据证实MT的有效性

MT的获益已在广泛的医疗保健系统中得到有效证实——临床试验包括来自西欧、美国、加拿大、韩国、澳大利亚和新西兰的9个国家[9,12-16,18,26,32,174,183,188,224]。2014年10月,在MR CLEAN临床试验结果公布以后[18],尽管有很多关于MT的临床试验提前结束[12-14,16,26],其实大多数试验已经积累了足够的数据来证明已经达到了有利于MT的预设的疗效终点[13,14,16]。而MT开始时间(>6小时)的试验规模较小,并且使用了不同的入选标准,而6小时以外的MT疗效不如6小时内相对明显。序贯试验表明,与单独药物治疗相比,MT治疗的患者预后的优势比没有变化[12,13,16,18,26,32,224]。

对试验数据的荟萃分析表明,尽管有降低20%的趋势,但MT并不具有显著的死亡率优势[225,226]。

MT的安全性

许多术中和术后并发症与MT相关[227],需要有效地将其最小化并设法使其获益最大化。总体而言,患者接受MT治疗出现并发症而形成后遗症的风险约为15%[9,12-16,18,26,32,188,224]。有些并发症危及生命,可能会延长重症监护和卒中病房的住院时间,而另一些并发症会增加费用并延误康复。某些并发症是可以预防的,而其他并发症的影响则可以通过早期发现和适当的管理而降到最低。神经介入医生需要了解与MT相关的危险因素、预防策略和并发症管理。神经介入医生需要了解危险因素、预防策略以及相关并发症的处理。然而,与取栓过程相关的发病率和死亡率几乎总是在30天内发生的,因此90天患者预后作为MT的净获益,这对其极为有利[227]。

不确定的领域

当前的荟萃分析极少包括有后循环 LVO 的患者。尽管在非随机研究中 MT 在后循环中的再通效果与前者相符，但在后循环卒中之中仍需证实其临床获益，并且正在进行试验。近期由于中国关于基底动脉闭塞取栓试验因跨组过多而导致提前中止了试验。相关信息已有提及但尚未正式公布，表明 MT 对 intention-to-treat 组并无获益，而对 as-treated 组有获益[227]。

需要进行进一步的试验来探索是否可以使用脑部影像学检查来筛选患者进行 MT 的延迟治疗，入院早期采用先进的脑部影像学检查是否会影响预后，临床实践中使用全身麻醉还是局部麻醉，MT 治疗发病前已残疾的患者是否有获益等[227,228]。

13. MT 的社区宣教

医疗专家和公共卫生官员需要制定卒中教育计划，重点关注症状，寻求急诊治疗和可用的卒中系统资源[229]。该计划应该面向社区内的所有人群，以符合他们的经济、社会和道德需要[230]。提高对卒中症状的认识对于寻求及时治疗至关重要[229]。与普通人群相比，社区少数人群对卒中的危险因素和症状的认识较低。因此，他们很少呼叫 EMS，从而会延误必要的治疗[231]。延误治疗会导致治疗效果下降，并使死亡率升高[232]。近几年，随着综合卒中治疗系统的建立，以及公共卒中教育的加强，IVT 和 MT 的例数明显增加。此外，应提高人们对周围可用急诊调度系统的认识，以缩短卒中发生时间到 EMS 到达的时间间隔[229]。EMS 的激活和卒中患者的转运与尽早到达（发病到入院时间 ≤ 3 小时）、更快的评估（入院到成像时间 ≤ 25 分钟）、更快的治疗转运（更多入院到穿刺时间 ≤ 60 分钟）、更多患者符合 MT 适应证和更多的患者接受静脉 rt-PA 治疗（67% vs 44%）独立相关[233]。

14. 机械取栓培训计划

EMS 培训、评估和管理

卒中治疗的时间窗很短。因此，EMS 专业人员应在快速诊断、评估、管理、治疗、分诊和快速运送卒中患者等方面训练有素并经验丰富[234]。患者预后改善已证实与 EMS 调度员和卒中评估和确诊的现场人员指导患者选择最合适的 TSC 有关[235,236]。洛杉矶院前卒中筛查 LAPSS、CPSS 和 MASS 对卒中评估的敏感性均超过 90%[237-240]。另一种筛查工具是"视力、失语和忽视"（VAN）评估，它无需评分系统即可评估神经血管功能，却已被证明可有效识别到院时出现 LVO 且严重程度超过 NIHSS ≥ 6 的卒中患者，是判定因卒中引起的损伤程度的最常用评估方法之一。它可以快速识别出适合进行血管内治疗的缺血性卒中患者和因接受脑部手术的高危脑出血患者[14,15]。与 NIHSS 和其他已建立的院前大血管闭塞筛查工具相比，它在院内也被证明是有效的[241]。实际上，尽管 VAN 和 NIHSS 量表均具有 100% 的敏感性，VAN 比 NIHSS ≥ 6 的工具具有更高的阳性预测值（分别为 74% 和 58%）和特异性（90% 和 74%）[242]。此外，VAN 的实施显著缩短了患者入院到实施 CTA 检查的时间 [77（±43）分钟 vs 27（±23）分钟，$P < 0.05$)][243]。

为了使急救医护人员对疑似 LVO 卒中的患者做好准备，EMS 需要向接收医院提供到达前的通知。事实上，这将使患者在 3 小时内可接受 IVT 的概率增加（82.8% vs 79.2%），到院 - 影像检查时间缩短（26 分钟 vs 31 分钟），入院 - 穿刺时间缩短（78 分钟 vs 80 分钟），症状出现 - 穿刺时间缩短（141 分钟 vs 145 分钟）[244]。此外，基于 EMS 对 LVO 卒中患者的诊断，可以将其运送到设备条件完善的高级卒中中心，这对患者的预后至关重要。

培训神经介入医生

MT 的操作医生必须具备相关技术的足够培训的经历和经验,包括基础培训和专业继续教育[245,246]。然而,只有少数医院能给医生提供 MT 培训。因此,建立专门的区域 TSC 十分有必要,以确保医生有足够的机械取栓手术量和操作经验[247]。

基线培训和资格

住院医师培训内容包括医师培训,在有执业认证的神经放射科医生、神经内科医生或神经外科医生的指导下,对 AIS 的诊断和管理,对脑动脉造影和神经影像学结果的解读,并最终获得技术专长。在其住院培训结束时,他们必须获得该领域的资质认证。随后,在高容量的中心和神经介入医生的监督下接受 AIS 的神经介入放射学专科培训,并将获得 AIS 特定的治疗经验,例如,如何克服具有挑战性的解剖结构以建立通路,在脑循环内如何使微导管到位,以及如何避免和处理介入并发症[245]。

医生资质的保持

卒中的治疗领域日新月异,因此,应要求医生每两年至少进行 16 个小时的卒中教育。此外,鼓励医生参加质量和改进监督项目。该项目将审查急性卒中介入性治疗质量并随访相关治疗结果[245,246]。

培训卒中治疗团队

卒中治疗的有效性是有时间依赖性的,已证明 4.5 小时时间窗外的 IVT 疗效会降低[175]。对于血管内治疗如 MT,已经表明了类似的时间依赖性[188]。AIS-LVO 的标准治疗方法是 IVT 联合 MT,能为患者带来更好的患者预后[248],但是这需要组建多学科卒中团队来实现。为了最大限度地减少治疗时间和非技术性错误,建议将仿真团队培训作为任何 TSC

的核心组成部分[249]。已经证实，基于仿真的干预措施可以将入院到穿刺时间中位数减少 12 分钟（IQR 29.8~60.0，n=122）到 31 分钟（IQR 240~420，n=112），并增加到院 30 分钟内 IVT 的患者数量（41.5%~59.6%，P<0.001））[250]。

15. 卒中取栓中心的发展

5 项多中心、前瞻性、随机、开放标签、盲态终点的临床试验表明，MT 治疗 AIS-LVO 患者具有显著的临床获益[10,14-16,18]。重要的是，这些试验是在高容量的卒中中心开展的，并且这些中心拥有经验丰富的卒中专家，因此有能力为患者提供复杂的治疗。医疗机构的卒中团队由急诊科医生、放射科医生、神经介入医生、神经科医生、神经重症医生、神经外科医生和接受过卒中培训的辅助人员组成。这些关键人员对取栓中心提供高效的治疗至关重要[10,14-16,18,251]。

2016 年，SVIN 提出了促进 LVO 卒中系统发展的建议，包括将 MT 作为一种治疗方法[251]。这些建议补充了对目前综合性卒中中心的资格要求，包括高患者容量、先进的影像能力、院后协调治疗、专门的神经重症监护、质量控制、参与卒中研究和汇报绩效指标等。SVIN 建议对这些标准进行如下补充。

高患者容量

高容量的治疗措施与患者的良好预后息息相关[252-255]。SVIN 建议需要每年应用 MT 治疗 25~30 例患者，CSC 的所有神经介入医生应每年至少完成 10 例 MT[251]。

先进的影像能力

推荐所有的 CSC 都具有能够治疗两名同时发生 LVO 卒中患者的能力；

因此需要神经介入专家和相关的辅助人员随叫随到、卒中介入手术室随时可用[251]。

院后协调治疗

推荐在 CSC 和康复中心之间建立一个监测和协调的系统，以确保后续的治疗。此类卒中后的治疗机构应获得卒中康复认证，工作人员应接受标准化的预后量表的培训[251]。

专门的神经重症监护病房和神经介入专家和神经外科管理

由于 AIS 卒中患者治疗管理的复杂性和潜在的并发症，由血管神经科医生和神经重症专家组成的多学科团队应随叫随到[251]。

同行评审过程

推荐目前建立的同行评审流程应纳入 MT 治疗 AIS-LVO 患者快速高效相关的绩效指标。English 等人[251]提供了这些指标的综合量表。

许多里程碑式临床研究有助于改进患者入院后的诊治流程系统，但入院前时间管理和根据患者症状严重程度分诊仍然是优化患者运输绩效指标的最重要因素[256]。更长的 DIDO 时间会对 LVO 卒中患者的预后产生不利的影响，这可能是发病–再通时间中单一最大的可控因素[257]。即使是高容量的初级卒中中心（PSC）在大城市的中心辐射圈中，由指定的 CSC 为 PSC 提供取栓技术支持仍有很长的 DIDO 时间（中位时间为 106 分钟）和转运时间（中位转运时间为 128 分钟）[258]。因此，推荐 DIDO 作为常规绩效指标并积极缩短。在 PSC 中，持续的质量改进流程已被证明可以将中位 DIDO 时间缩短到少于 60 分钟[259]。在设计个性化院前转运策略时，需要考虑 LVO 的风险，在农村或城市地区的驾车时间和医院的工作流程时间，以实现 AIS 患者获得最佳预后[260]。

急性卒中机械取栓：现状与经验

院间转运的优点和缺点

多项里程碑式的研究已经证实动脉内取栓能使患者获益[10,14-16,18,25]；因此，美国心脏学会和美国卒中学会（AHA/ASA）更新的2013年的指南，以反映改善卒中治疗系统的必要性，包括院前分诊、院间转诊和PSC、CSC的认证[261]。这些推荐在最新的2019年的ASA指南中保持不变，继续强调院前治疗、急诊评估、静脉溶栓和动脉取栓治疗方法和院内管理的重要性。院间转运到能够行血管内治疗的中心提供机械取栓治疗。然而，取栓前的院间转运可延误治疗并且对前循环AIS-LVO患者的预后有不利的影响[262]。这些结果与荷兰的一项研究结果一致，但荷兰卒中中心之间距离相对较近[263]。现场识别为LVO后并且直接收入能行血管内治疗的CSC的患者往往有较好的预后[264,265]。因此，EMS应该绕过附近的PSC并直接将患者转运到CSC。为了缩短转运时间，所有的PSC都应该开展MT[266]。

无效转院的原因

2009—2014年，缺血性卒中的院间转运增长了33%，MT的需求量加大[267]。法国的一项研究证实，45%的因MT而转院是无效的患者最终未能接受介入治疗，可能是因为转院期间血管闭塞增加导致临床症状恶化[268]。院间转运后未行MT的主要原因包括：梗死已形成、LVO血管再通和临床症状得到改善[269]。此外，院间转运过程中由于ASPECTS评分降低，约1/3的患者不适合行MT[41,42]。

影响血管内治疗延误的因素包括：最早发现人的识别、EMS效率、院间转运、通知血管内治疗团队和流程内的延误[270]。通过较高的侧支评分、较高的NIHSS评分和来自初级转诊中心的CTA影像，可独立预测转运后患者接受MT的概率[43,44]。

转运过程中的延误

DIDO时间是发病到再通时间中单一最大可控的因素，较长的DIDO时间可以给LVO-AIS患者的预后带来不利影响[257]。对美国的两家偏远地区大型卒中远程会诊系统的DIDO时间分析表明，院间转运前行CTA检查可增加取栓中心患者入院-股动脉穿刺时间[271]。即使是对处在大城市的中心辐射圈内高容量的PSC来说，DIDO时间和从PSC到CSC之间的转运时间也是较长的[258]。

医院工作流程的质量改进

通过质量改进可改善患者在较远的CSC再灌注治疗的延迟[272]。许多里程碑式的研究也有助于改善患者直接入院后的院内工作流程，但是根据区域卒中救护系统的真实数据，院前时间管理和分诊仍是优化患者运输绩效指标最重要的因素[18]。优化院内治疗流程对于预防转院的延误和MT的相关延误至关重要[49]。2017年SVIN的一篇报道建议，由于LVO卒中患者发病和死亡的风险不断攀升，需尽快实现再灌注，这取决于优化医院的诊治流程[50]。标准化PSC方案的一些特性包括尽早通知CSC、云数据共享和到院时的CTA，这与改善LVO卒中患者的预后相关[45,51]。在一项单中心研究中，规范了治疗急诊LVO的医疗方案和流程后，手术时间如穿刺-再通的总时间从68.2分钟降到37.0分钟[52,273]。对卒中患者从PSC转运到CSC决定进行详细的系统分类，可以帮助减少患者不适当的转运并改善预后[53]。

移动诊疗模式

卒中治疗的移动诊疗模式，是由可移动的卒中介入小组在PSC提供介入治疗，这比患者在最近的医院行血管内治疗的逐级转运模式快了79分钟（$P<0.0001$）。因此，这种模式是在城市中院间转运的一种潜在替代

方案[274]。

卒中远程会诊的选项

卒中远程会诊是一种专门从事卒中诊疗的专家通过技术手段帮助其他地区的卒中患者进行治疗的方法，提高了卒中患者的 MT 治疗率，减少了转院的必要性[274]。夏威夷的卒中远程会诊项目每年咨询的次数从 2012 年的 11 次增加到了 2016 年的 203 次。因此，越来越多的血管再通的手术在神经学科较弱的医院开展，这是一种解决医疗资源不平均的潜在方案[55]。

直升机紧急医疗服务

直升机紧急医疗服务（HEMS）的作用需要进一步明确，以便在转运过程中提供更好的辅助治疗，并消除患者基于地理位置的限制接受取栓治疗的差异[275]。在美国，需要解决的一个差异是西班牙裔卒中患者与非西班牙裔白人卒中患者相比，使用 HEMS 的情况不同，这降低或消除了患者及时接受 MT 的概率[276]。

B. 团队培训原则

2016 年	A Community-Engaged Assessment of Barriers and Facilitators to Rapid Stroke Treatment https://www.ncbi.nlm.nih.gov/pubmed/27545591
2007–2012 年	Heart Disease and Stroke in Illinois: Now is the time for Public Health Action http://www.idph.state.il.us/heartstroke/state_plan_book2.pdf
2013 年	American Heart Association Guide for Improving Cardiovascular Health at the Community Level: A Statement for Public Health Practitioners, Healthcare Providers, and Health Policy Makers from the American Heart Association Expert Panel on Population and Prevention Science https://www.ahajournals.org/doi/full/10.1161/cir.0b013e31828f8a94
2010 年	A Population-Based Policy and Systems Change Approach to Prevent and Control Hypertension. https://www.ncbi.nlm.nih.gov/books/NBK220093/

C. 基本的/主要的预防原则

2019 年	Stroke Prevention https://emedicine.medscape.com/article/323662-overview
2019 年	Guidelines for the Early Management of Patients with Acute Ischemic Stroke: 2019 Update to the 2018 Guidelines for the Early Management of Acute Ischemic Stroke: A Guideline for Healthcare Professionals From the American Heart Association/American Stroke Association https://pubmed.ncbi.nlm.nih.gov/31662037-guidelines-for-the-early-management-of-patients-with-acute-ischemic-stroke-2019-up-date-to-the-2018-guidelines-for-the-early-management-of-acute-ischemic-stroke-a-guide-line-for-healthcare-professionals-from-the-american-heart-associationamerican-stroke-association/?from_term=2018+Guidelines+for+the+Early+Management+of+Patients+With+Acute+Ischemic+Stroke%3A+A+Guideline+for+Healthcare+-Professionals+From+the+American+Heart+Association%2FAmerican+Stroke+Association&from_page=1&from_pos=2
2018 年	2018 Guidelines for the Early Management of Patients with Acute Ischemic Stroke: A Guideline for Healthcare Professionals from the American Heart Association/American Stroke Association https://www.bmc.org/sites/default/fles/Patient_Care/Specialty_Care/Stroke_and_Cerebro-vascular_Center/Medical_Professionals/Protocols/2018%20AHA%20Ischemic%20Stroke%20Guideline%20Update%202018.pdf
2018 年	Recent Advances in Primary and Secondary Prevention of Atherosclerotic Stroke https://www.j-stroke.org/journal/view.php?number=225

附 录

2017 年	Blood Pressure Reduction and Secondary Stroke Prevention: A Systematic Review and Metaregression Analysis of Randomized Clinical Trials https://pubmed.ncbi.nlm.nih.gov/27802419-blood-pressure-reduction-and-secondary-stroke-prevention-a-systematic-review-and-metaregression-analysis-of-randomzed-clinical-trials/?from_term=Current+Recom-mendations+for+Secondary+Stroke+Prevention&-from_pos=6
2016 年	Stroke Prevention https://www.ncbi.nlm.nih.gov/pubmed/27816341
2014 年	Guidelines for the prevention of stroke in patients with stroke and transient ischemic attack: a guideline for healthcare professionals from the American Heart Association/American Stroke Association https://www.ncbi.nlm.nih.gov/pubmed/24788967
2014 年	Guidelines for the prevention of stroke in women: a statement for healthcare professionals from the American Heart Association/American Stroke Association https://www.ahajournals.org/doi/abs/10.1161/01.str.0000442009.06663.48
2014 年	Guidelines for the Primary Prevention of Stroke: A Statement for Healthcare Professionals From the American Heart Association/American Stroke Association https://www.ahajournals.org/doi/10.1161/STR.0000000000000046
2008 年	Update to the AHA/ASA recommendations for the prevention of stroke in patients with stroke and transient ischemic attack https://www.ahajournals.org/doi/abs/10.1161/strokeaha.107.189063

D. 急诊处理原则

2018 年	2018 guidelines for the early management of patients with actue ischemic stroke: a guideline for healthcare professionals from the American Heart Association/American Stroke Association https://www.ahajournals.org/doi/abs/10.1161/STR.0000000000000158
2013 年	Guidelines for the early management of patients with acute ischemic stroke: a guideline for healthcare professionals from the American Heart Association/American Stroke Association https://www.ahajournals.org/doi/abs/10.1161/str.0b013e318284056a
2007 年	EMS management of acute stroke--prehospital triage (resource document to NAEMSP position statement) https://www.tandfonline.com/doi/abs/10.1080/10903120701347844
2005 年	Recommendations for the Establishment of Stroke Systems of Care: Recommendations from the American Stroke Association's Task Force on the Development of StrokeSystems https://www.ahajournals.org/doi/full/10.1161/01.cir.0000154252.62394.1e

E. 以医院为中心的急性卒中管理原则

2019 年	Recommendations for the Establishment of Stroke Systems of Care: A 2019 Update https://www.ncbi.nlm.nih.gov/pubmed/?term=Recommendations+for+the+Establishment+of+Stroke+Systems+of+Care%3A+A+2019+Up-date
2019 年	Guidelines for the Early Management of Patients with Acute Ischemic Stroke: 2019 Update to the 2018 Guidelines for the Early Management of Acute Ischemic Stroke: A Guideline for Healthcare Professionals from the American Heart Association/American Stroke Association https://www.ncbi.nlm.nih.gov/pubmed/31662037

2019年	Management of Acute Ischemic Stroke: a Review of Pertinent Guideline Updates https://www.uspharmacist.com/article/management-of-acute-ischemic-stroke-a-review-of-pertinent-guideline-updates
2019年	Ischemic Stroke: Management by the Nurse Practitioner https://www.npjournal.org/article/S1555-4155(18)30500-2/fulltext
2019年	Society of Interventional Radiology Training Guidelines for Endovascular Stroke Treatment DOI: https://doi.org/10.1016/j.jvir.2019.08.018
2019年	2019 Update of the Korean Clinical Practice Guidelines of Stroke for Endovascular Recanalization Therapy in Patients with Acute Ischemic Stroke https://doi.org/10.5853/jos.2019.00024
2019年	European Stroke Organisation (ESO) – European Society for Minimally Invasive Neurological Therapy (ESMINT) Guidelines on Mechanical Thrombectomy in Acute Ischemic Stroke https://www.ncbi.nlm.nih.gov/pubmed/30808653
2018年	2018 Guidelines for the Early Management of Patients with Acute Ischemic Stroke: A Guideline for Healthcare Professionals from the American Heart Association/American Stroke Association https://www.ncbi.nlm.nih.gov/pubmed/29367334
2018年	Canadian Stroke Best Practice Recommendations for Acute Stroke Management: Prehospital, Emergency Department, and Acute Inpatient Stroke Care, 6th Edition, Update 2018 https://www.ncbi.nlm.nih.gov/pubmed/30021503

2018 年	Get with The Guidelines – Stroke Clinical Tools https://www.heart.org/en/professional/quality-improvement/get-with-the-guidelines/get-with-the-guidelines-stroke/get-with-the-guidelines-stroke-clinical-tools
2018 年	Diagnosis and Management of Acute Ischemic Stroke https://doi.org/10.1016/j.mayocp.2018.02.013
2018 年	TREATMENT OF ACUTE ISCHEMIC STROKE https://www.va.gov/vhapublications/ViewPublication.asp?pub_ID=6438
2018 年	Complications of endovascular treatment for acute ischemic stroke: Prevention and management https://www.ncbi.nlm.nih.gov/pubmed/29171362
2018 年	International Comparison of Patient Characteristics and Quality of Care for Ischemic Stroke: Analysis of the China National Stroke Registry and the American Heart Association Get With The Guidelines--Stroke Program. https://www.ncbi.nlm.nih.gov/pubmed/30371291
2018 年	Multisociety Consensus Quality Improvement Revised Consensus Statement for Endovascular Therapy of Acute Ischemic Stroke https://www.ncbi.nlm.nih.gov/pubmed/29478797
2018 年	The organisation of the acute ischemic stroke management: key notes of the Italian Neurological Society and of the Italian Stroke Organization https://www.ncbi.nlm.nih.gov/pubmed/29181655
2018 年	Standards of Practice in Acute Ischemic Stroke Intervention: International Recommendations https://www.ncbi.nlm.nih.gov/pubmed/30442688

2017 年	A systematic comparison of key features of ischemic stroke prevention guidelines in low- and middle-income *vs* high-income countries https://www.ncbi.nlm.nih.gov/pubmed/28008094
2017 年	Differences in Acute Ischemic Stroke Quality of Care and Outcomes by Primary Stroke Center Certifcation Organization https://www.ncbi.nlm.nih.gov/pubmed/28008094
2017 年	Brazilian guidelines for endovascular treatment of patients with acute ischemic stroke https://www.ncbi.nlm.nih.gov/pubmed/28099563
2017 年	The Chinese Stroke Association scientifc statement: intravenous thrombolysis in acute ischaemic stroke https://www.ncbi.nlm.nih.gov/pubmed/28989804
2016 年	Guidelines for Adult Stroke Rehabilitation and Recovery: A Guideline for Healthcare Professionals From the American Heart Association/American Stroke Association https://www.ncbi.nlm.nih.gov/pubmed/27145936
2016 年	Diagnosis and Initial Treatment of Ischemic Stroke https://www.icsi.org/wp-content/uploads/2019/01/Stroke.pdf
2016 年	Quality Improvement in Acute Ischemic Stroke Care in Taiwan: The Breakthrough Collaborative in Stroke https://doi.org/10.1371/journal.pone.0160426
2016 年	Training Guidelines for Endovascular Ischemic Stroke Intervention: An International multi-society consensus document https://www.ncbi.nlm.nih.gov/pubmed/26888954

2015 年	Canadian Association of Emergency Physicians position statement on acute ischemic stroke https://www.ncbi.nlm.nih.gov/pubmed/26120643
2010 年	Acute Stroke Practice Guidelines for Inpatient Management of Ischemic Stroke and Transient Ischemic Attack (TIA) https://www.heart.org/idc/groups/heart-public/@private/@wcm/@hcm/documents/downloadable/ucm_309996.pdf

F. 二级预防及急性期后管理原则

2020 年	Overview of secondary prevention of ischemic stroke https://www.uptodate.com/contents/over-view-of-secondary-prevention-of-ischemic-stroke
2019 年	Recommendations for the Establishment of Stroke Systems of Care: A 2019 Update. https://www.ahajournals.org/doi/10.1161/STR.0000000000000173
2019 年	Ischemic Stroke: Management by the Nurse Practitioner DOI: https://doi.org/10.1016/j.nurpra.2018.07.019
2005 年	Recommendations for the Establishment of Stroke Systems of Care: Recommendations from the American Stroke Association's Task Force on the Development of StrokeSystems https://www.ahajournals.org/doi/full/10.1161/01.cir.0000154252.62394.1e

2019年	Antithrombotic treatment for secondary prevention of stroke and other thromboembolic events in patients with stroke or transient ischemic attack and non-valvular atrial fbrillation: A European Stroke Organisation guideline https://journals.sagepub.com/doi/full/10.1177/2396987319841187
2019年	Secondary prevention of stroke in patients with atrial fbrillation: factors infuencing the prescription of oral anticoagulation at discharge https://www.ncbi.nlm.nih.gov/pubmed/31662037
2018年	2018 Guidelines for the Early Management of Patients with Acute Ischemic Stroke: A Guideline for Healthcare Professionals from the American Heart Association/American Stroke Association https://www.ncbi.nlm.nih.gov/pubmed/29367334
2018年	Canadian stroke best practice consensus statement: Secondary stroke prevention during pregnancy https://www.ncbi.nlm.nih.gov/pubmed/29171360
2018年	Recent Advances in Primary and Secondary Prevention of Atherosclerotic Stroke https://www.j-stroke.org/journal/view.php?number=225
2017年	Canadian stroke best practice recommendations: Secondary prevention of stroke, sixth edition practice guidelines, update 2017 https://www.ncbi.nlm.nih.gov/pubmed/29171361 https://journals.sagepub.com/doi/full/10.1177/1747493017743062
2017年	Secondary Prevention of Stroke: 6th Edition 2017 UPDATE https://www.strokebestpractices.ca/recommendations/secondary-prevention-of-stroke

2016 年	Stroke and Stroke Rehabilitation: Quality Measurement Set Update
	https://www.aan.com/siteassets/home-page/policy-and-guidelines/quality/quality-measures/15strokeandrehabmeasureset_pg.pdf
2016 年	Quality-Based Procedures: Clinical Handbook for Stroke (Acute and Postacute)
	http://health.gov.on.ca/en/pro/programs/ecfa/docs/qbp_stroke.pdf
2016 年	National clinical guideline for stroke SSNAP
	https://www.strokeaudit.org/SupportFiles/Documents/Guidelines/2016-National-Clinical-Guide-line-for-Stroke-5t-(1).aspx
2016 年	Guidelines for Management of Hyperlipidemia: Implications for Treatment of Patients with Stroke Secondary to Atherosclerotic Disease
	https://www.ncbi.nlm.nih.gov/pubmed/26838351
2016 年	Secondary Prevention of Stroke
	http://www.ebrsr.com/sites/default/fles/Chapter%208_Secondary%20Prevention%20of%20Stroke.pdf
2015 年	Quality-Based Procedures: Clinical Handbook for Stroke (Acute and Postacute)
	http://www.hqontario.ca/Portals/0/Documents/evidence/clinical-handbooks/community-stroke-20151802-en.pdf
2015 年	Antithrombotic Management of Patients with Nonvalvular Atrial Fibrillation and Ischemic Stroke or Transient Ischemic Attack: Executive Summary of the Korean Clinical Practice Guidelines for Stroke
	https://www.ncbi.nlm.nih.gov/pubmed/26060808

附 录

2014 年	Guidelines for the prevention of stroke in patients with stroke and transient ischemic attack: a guideline for healthcare professionals from the American Heart Association/American Stroke Association. https://www.ncbi.nlm.nih.gov/pubmed/24788967
2014 年	2014 Chinese guidelines for secondary prevention of ischemic stroke and transient ischemic attack. https://www.ncbi.nlm.nih.gov/pubmed/28381199
2014 年	Canadian Stroke Best Practice Recommendations: secondary prevention of stroke guidelines, update 2014. https://www.ncbi.nlm.nih.gov/pubmed/25535808
2013 年	Key articles and guidelines in the acute management and secondary prevention of ischemic stroke https://www.ncbi.nlm.nih.gov/pubmed/23401103
2012 年	Stroke Clinical Care Programme Model of Care-HSE https://www.hse.ie/eng/services/publications/clinical-strategy-and-programmes/stroke-model-of-care.pdf
2012 年	Model of Stroke Care 2012 https://ww2.health.wa.gov.au/~/media/Files/Corpo-rate/general%20documents/Health%20Networks/Neurosciences%20and%20the%20Senses/Model-of-Stroke-Care.pdf
2012 年	Chinese guidelines for the secondary prevention of ischemic stroke and transient ischemic attack 2010. https://www.ncbi.nlm.nih.gov/pubmed/22313945
2012 年	Inclusion of stroke in cardiovascular risk prediction instruments: a statement for healthcare professionals from the American Heart Association/American Stroke Association. https://www.ncbi.nlm.nih.gov/pubmed/22627990

2011 年	AHA/ASA Guidelines on Prevention of Recurrent Stroke https://www.aafp.org/afp/2011/0415/p993.html
2011 年	Subacute Management of Ischemic Stroke https://www.aafp.org/afp/2011/1215/p1383.html
2010 年	New Zealand Clinical Guidelines for Stroke Management 2010 https://www.health.govt.nz/system/fles/documents/publications/nzclinicalguidelinesstrokemanage-ment2010activecontents.pdf
2010 年	Clinical Guidelines for Stroke Management 2010 https://extranet.who.int/ncdccs/Data/AUS_D1_Clinical%20Guidelines%20for%20Stroke%20Management.pdf
2010 年	Management of Stroke Rehabilitation https://www.healthquality.va.gov/stroke/str_full_220.pdf
2010 年	Current Recommendations for Secondary Stroke Prevention https://www.uspharmacist.com/article/current-recommendations-for-secondary-stroke-prevention
2009 年	Stroke and Transient Ischaemic Attacks – Ministry of Health https://www.moh.gov.sg/docs/librariesprovider4/guidelines/cpg_stroke-and-transient-ischaemic-attacks.pdf

G. 卒中康复原则

2019 年	Evidence-Based Guidelines and Clinical Pathways in Stroke Rehabilitation-An International Perspective https://www.ncbi.nlm.nih.gov/pubmed/?term=Evidence-Based+Guidelines+and+Clinical+Pathways+in+Stroke+Rehabilitation%E2%80%94An+International+Perspective

2019 年	The Management of Stroke Rehabilitation: A Synopsis of the 2019 U.S. Department of Veterans Affairs and U.S. Department of Defense Clinical Practice Guideline
	https://www.ncbi.nlm.nih.gov/pubmed/31739317
2019 年	Assessment and Management of Patients at Risk for Suicide: Synopsis of the 2019 U.S. Department of Veterans Affairs and U.S. Department of Defense Clinical Practice Guidelines
	https://www.ncbi.nlm.nih.gov/pubmed/31450237
2019 年	VA/DoD CLINICAL PRACTICE GUIDELINE FOR THE MANAGEMENT OF STROKE REHABILITATION
	https://www.healthquality.va.gov/guidelines/Rehab/stroke/VADoDStrokeRehabCPGFinal8292019.pdf
2019 年	Stroke rehabilitation: therapy
	https://pathways.nice.org.uk/pathways/stroke
2019 年	The Subacute Rehabilitation of Childhood Stroke, Clinical Guideline 2019
	https://informme.org.au/en/Guidelines/Child-hood-stroke-guidelines
2019 年	Clinical Practice Guideline for Cardiac Rehabilitation in Korea.
	https://www.ncbi.nlm.nih.gov/pubmed/31404368
	https://www.ncbi.nlm.nih.gov/pubmed/31311260
2019 年	Clinical Practice Guideline for Cardiac Rehabilitation in Korea: Recommendations for Cardiac Rehabilitation and Secondary Prevention after Acute Coronary Syndrome.
	https://www.ncbi.nlm.nih.gov/pubmed/31646772
2018 年	Guidelines for Adult Stroke Rehabilitation and Recovery
	https://www.ncbi.nlm.nih.gov/pubmed/?term=JAMA+Guidelines+for+Adult+Stroke+Rehabilitation+and+Recovery

2018 年	Elderly Stroke Rehabilitation: Overcoming the Complications and Its Associated Challenges https://www.hindawi.com/journals/cggr/2018/9853837/
2018 年	Systematic review of clinical practice guidelines to identify recommendations for rehabilitation after stroke and other acquired brain injuries https://www.ncbi.nlm.nih.gov/pubmed/29490958
2018 年	Korean Clinical Practice Guidelines for Aneurysmal Subarachnoid Hemorrhage. https://www.ncbi.nlm.nih.gov/pubmed/29526058
2017 年	Stroke Rehabilitation: Current American Stroke Association Guidelines, Care, and Implications for Practice https://www.ncbi.nlm.nih.gov/pmc/articles/PMC6143585/
2017 年	Stroke in childhood – clinical guideline for diagnosis, management and rehabilitation https://www.rcpch.ac.uk/resources/stroke-childhood-clinical-guideline-diagnosis-management-rehabilitation#fullclinicalguideline
2016 年	Guidelines for Adult Stroke Rehabilitation and Recovery: A Guideline for Healthcare Professionals from the American Heart Association/American Stroke Association https://www.ncbi.nlm.nih.gov/pubmed/27145936
2016 年	EVIDENCE-BASED REVIEW OF STROKE REHABILITATION (18th Edition) http://www.ebrsr.com/sites/default/fles/documents/v18-SREBR-ExecutiveSummary-2.pdf

附 录

2016 年	Clinical Practice Guideline for Stroke Rehabilitation in Korea 2016 https://synapse.koreamed.org/Synapse/Data/PDF-Data/0176BN/bn-10-e11.pdf
2016 年	2016 European Guidelines on cardiovascular disease prevention in clinical practice: The Sixth Joint Task Force of the European Society of Cardiology and Other Societies on Cardiovascular Disease Prevention in Clinical Practice (constituted by representatives of 10 societies and by invited experts)Developed with the special contribution of the European Association for Cardiovascular Prevention & Rehabilitation (EACPR). https://www.ncbi.nlm.nih.gov/pubmed/27222591
2016 年	2016 European Guidelines on cardiovascular disease prevention in clinical practice: The Sixth Joint Task Force of the European Society of Cardiology and Other Societies on Cardiovascular Disease Prevention in Clinical Practice (constituted by representatives of 10 societies and by invited experts) Developed with the special contribution of the European Association for Cardiovascular Prevention & Rehabilitation (EACPR). https://www.ncbi.nlm.nih.gov/pubmed/27664503
2016 年	Assessing and treating pain associated with stroke, multiple sclerosis, cerebral palsy, spinal cord injury and spasticity. Evidence and recommendations from theItalian Consensus Conference on Pain in Neurorehabilitation https://www.ncbi.nlm.nih.gov/pubmed/27579581
2016 年	Canadian Stroke Best Practice Recommendations: Managing transitions of care following Stroke, Guidelines Update 2016. https://www.ncbi.nlm.nih.gov/pubmed/27443991
2015 年	Stroke Rehabilitation	Canadian Stroke Best Practices https://www.strokebestpractices.ca/recommendations/stroke-rehabilitation

2015 年	Canadian stroke best practice recommendations: Stroke rehabilitation practice guidelines, update 2015 https://www.ncbi.nlm.nih.gov/pubmed/27079654
2015 年	Guidelines for the Management of Spontaneous Intracerebral Hemorrhage Guidelines for the Management of Spontaneous Intracerebral Hemorrhage
2014 年	Physical activity and exercise recommendations for stroke survivors: a statement for healthcare professionals from the American Heart Association/American Stroke Association https://www.ncbi.nlm.nih.gov/pubmed/24846875
2014 年	Best practice guidelines for stroke in Cameroon: An innovative and participatory knowledge translation project https://www.ncbi.nlm.nih.gov/pubmed/28729996
2013 年	Clinical Guideline on Stroke Rehabilitation https://extranet.who.int/ncdccs/Data/MNG_D1_2.%20Rehabilitation%20guideline%20of%20Stroke.pdf
2013 年	Stroke rehabilitation in adults: Clinical guideline [CG162] https://www.nice.org.uk/guidance/cg162
2012 年	Rehabilitation for Cerebrovascular Disease: Current and new methods in Japan https://www.ncbi.nlm.nih.gov/pubmed/25237224
2011 年	VII. Rehabilitation https://www.ncbi.nlm.nih.gov/pubmed/21835355
2011 年	The South African guideline for the management of ischemic stroke and transient ischemic attack: recommendations for a resource-constrained health care setting https://www.ncbi.nlm.nih.gov/pubmed/21745347

2010 年	Clinical Guidelines for Stroke Management 2010- PEDro https://www.pedro.org.au/wp-content/uploads/CPG_stroke.pdf
2010 年	Pathway for Stroke Rehabilitation https://www.sahealth.sa.gov.au/wps/wcm/connect/dd39a9804b32fb628730afe79043faf0/Stroke+Rehabilitation+Pathway.pdf?MOD=AJPERES&CACHEID=ROOTWORKSPACE-dd39a9804b32f-b628730afe79043faf0-mMz0iEE
2010 年	Management of patients with stroke: Rehabilitation, prevention and management ofcomplications, and discharge planning https://www.sign.ac.uk/assets/sign118.pdf
2010 年	Comprehensive overview of nursing and interdisciplinary rehabilitation care of the stroke patient: a scientifc statement from the American Heart Association https://www.ncbi.nlm.nih.gov/pubmed/20813995
2009 年	A review of the evidence for the use of telemedicine within stroke systems of care: a scientifc statement from the American Heart Association/ American Stroke Association. https://www.ncbi.nlm.nih.gov/pubmed/19423852

H. 姑息治疗及临终关怀原则

2018 年	Canadian Stroke Best Practice Recommendations for Acute Stroke Management: Prehospital, Emergency Department, and Acute Inpatient Stroke Care, 6th Edition, Update 2018. https://www.ncbi.nlm.nih.gov/pubmed/30021503

2016 年	Palliative Care and Cardiovascular Disease and Stroke: A Policy Statementfrom the American Heart Association/American Stroke Association. https://www.ncbi.nlm.nih.gov/pubmed/27503067
2014 年	Palliative and end-of-life care in stroke: a statement for healthcare professionals from the American Heart Association/American Stroke Association. https://www.ncbi.nlm.nih.gov/pubmed/24676781
2012 年	National clinical guideline for stroke: Fourth Edition http://citeseerx.ist.psu.edu/viewdoc/download?-doi=10.1.1.476.6093&rep=rep1&type=pdf
2012 年	Symptomatic and palliative care for stroke survivors. https://www.ncbi.nlm.nih.gov/pubmed/22258916

I. 持续治疗改进原则

2018 年	Multisociety Consensus Quality Improvement Revised Consensus Statement for Endovascular Therapy of Acute Ischemic Stroke: From the American Association of Neurological Surgeons (AANS), American Society of Neuroradiology (ASNR), Cardiovascular and Interventional Radiology Society of Europe (CIRSE), Canadian Interventional Radiology Association (CIRA), Congress of Neurological Surgeons (CNS), European Society of Minimally Invasive Neurological Therapy (ESMINT), European Society of Neuroradiology (ESNR), European Stroke Organization (ESO), Society for Cardiovascular Angiography and Interventions (SCAI), Society of Interventional Radiology (SIR), Society of NeuroInterventional Surgery (SNIS), and World Stroke Organization (WSO). https://www.ncbi.nlm.nih.gov/pubmed/29478797

2017 年	Stroke care quality in China: Substantial improvement, and a huge challenge and opportunity. https://www.ncbi.nlm.nih.gov/pubmed/?term=Stroke+care+quality+in+China%3A+Substantial+improvement%2C+and+a+huge+challenge+and+opportunity
2017 年	Standards for providing safe acute ischaemic stroke thrombectomy services (September 2015). https://www.ncbi.nlm.nih.gov/pubmed/27974152
2016 年	Quality Improvement in Acute Ischemic Stroke Care in Taiwan: The Breakthrough Collaborative in Stroke. https://www.ncbi.nlm.nih.gov/pubmed/?term=Quality+improvement+in+acute+ischemic+stroke+-care+in+Taiwan%3A+the+Breakthrough+Collaborative+in+Stroke
2016 年	The Danish Stroke Registry. https://www.ncbi.nlm.nih.gov/pubmed/27843349

参考文献

1. Lopez AD, Mathers CD, Ezzati M, et al. Global and regional burden of disease and risk factors, 2001: systematic analysis of population health data. Lancet,2006,367(9524):1747-1757.
2. Warlow CP. Epidemiology of stroke. Lancet,1998,352 (Suppl 3):SIII1-4.
3. Mozaffarian D, Benjamin EJ, Go AS, et al. Heart disease and stroke statistics-2015 update: a report from the American Heart Association. Circulation,2015,131(4):e29-322.
4. Donkor ES. Stroke in the 21(st) Century: A Snapshot of the Burden, Epidemiology, and Quality of Life. Stroke Res Treat,2018,2018:3238165.
5. Collaborators GS. Global, regional and national burden of stroke, 1990-2016: a systematic analysis for the Global Burden of Disease Study 2016. Lancet Neurol,2019,18(5):439-458.
6. Saver JL. Time is brain-quantified. Stroke,2006,37(1):263-266.
7. Goyal M, Almekhlafi M, Dippel DW, et al. Rapid alteplase administration improves functional outcomes in patients with stroke due to large vessel occlusions. Stroke,2019,50(3):645-651.
8. Robinson DJ. Should physicians give t-PA to patients with acute ischemic stroke? For: thrombolytics in stroke: whose risk is it anyway? West J Med,2000,173(3):148-149.
9. Albers GW, Marks MP, Kemp S, et al. Thrombectomy for stroke at 6 to 16 hours with selection by perfusion imaging. N Engl J Med, 2018,378(8):708-718.
10. Berkhemer OA, Fransen PS, Beumer D, et al. A randomized trial of intraarterial treatment for acute ischemic stroke. N Engl J Med, 2015,372(1):11-20.
11. Campbell BCV, Mitchell PJ, Churilov L, et al. Endovascular thrombectomy for ischemic stroke increases disability-free survival, quality of life, and life expectancy and reduces cost. Front Neuro,2017,8:657.

参考文献

12. Khoury NN, Darsaut TE, Ghostine J, et al. Endovascular thrombectomy and medical therapy versus medical therapy alone in acute stroke: A randomized care trial. J Neuroradiol,2017,44(3):198-202.

13. Mocco J, Zaidat OO, von Kummer R, et al. Aspiration thrombectomy after intravenous alteplase versus intravenous alteplase alone. Stroke,2016,47(9):2331-2338.

14. Campbell BC, Mitchell PJ, Kleinig TJ, et al. Endovascular therapy for ischemic stroke with perfusion-imaging selection. N Engl J Med,2015,372(11):1009-1018.

15. Goyal M, Demchuk AM, Menon BK, et al. Randomized assessment of rapid endovascular treatment of ischemic stroke. N Engl J Med,2015,372(11):1019-1030.

16. Saver JL, Goyal M, Bonafe A, et al. Stent-retriever thrombectomy after intravenous t-PA *vs* t-PA alone in stroke. N Engl J Med,2015,372(24):2285-2295.

17. Munich SA, Mokin M, Snyder KV, et al. Guest Editorial: An Update on Stroke Intervention. Neurosurgery,2015,77(3):313-320.

18. Jovin TG, Chamorro A, Cobo E, et al. Thrombectomy within 8 hours after symptom onset in ischemic stroke. N Engl J Med,2015,372(24):2296-2306.

19. Alawieh A, Vargas J, Fargen KM, et al. Impact of Procedure Time on Outcomes of Thrombectomy for Stroke. J Am Coll Cardiol,2019,73(8):879-890.

20. Shireman TI, Wang K, Saver JL, et al. Cost-Effectiveness of solitaire stent retriever thrombectomy for acute ischemic stroke: results from the swift-prime trial (solitaire with the intention for thrombectomy as primary endovascular treatment for acute ischemic stroke). Stroke,2017,48(2):379-387.

21. McCarthy DJ, Diaz A, Sheinberg DL, et al. Long-Term outcomes of mechanical thrombectomy for stroke: a meta-analysis. Scientific World Journal,2019,2019:7403104.

22. Luby M, Warach SJ, Albers GW, et al. Identification of imaging selection patterns in acute ischemic stroke patients and the influence on treatment and clinical trial enrollment decision making. Int J Stroke,2016,11(2):180-190.

23. Mullen MT, Branas CC, Kasner SE, et al. Optimization modeling to maximize population access to comprehensive stroke centers. Neurology,2015,84(12):1196-1205.

24. Mullen MT, Wiebe DJ, Bowman A, et al. Disparities in accessibility of certified primary stroke centers. Stroke,2014,45(11):3381-3388.

25. Jovin TG, Nogueira RG, Investigators D. Thrombectomy 6 to 24 Hours after stroke. N Engl J Med,2018,378(12):1161-1162.

26. Nogueira RG, Jadhav AP, Haussen DC, et al. Thrombectomy 6 to 24 hours after stroke with a mismatch between deficit and infarct. N Engl J Med,2018,378(1):11-21.
27. Gorelick PB. Primary and comprehensive stroke centers: history, value and certification criteria. J Stroke,2013,15(2):78-89.
28. Eurek A. SVIN announces 'Stroke: Mission thrombectomy 2020': An initiative to reduce disability from stroke worldwide Web site. https://www.eurekalert.org/pub_releases/2016-11/lpl-sa112116.php. Published 2016. Updated 21 Nov 2016. Accessed 31 Dec 2019.
29. Benjamin EJ, Blaha MJ, Chiuve SE, et al. Heart disease and stroke statistics-2017 update: a report from the american heart association. Circulation,2017,135(10):e146-e603.
30. Feigin VL, Lawes CM, Bennett DA, et al. Stroke epidemiology: a review of population-based studies of incidence, prevalence, and case-fatality in the late 20th century. Lancet Neurol,2003,2(1):43-53.
31. Ovbiagele B, Goldstein LB, Higashida RT, et al. Forecasting the future of stroke in the United States: a policy statement from the American Heart Association and American Stroke Association. Stroke,2013,44(8):2361-2375.
32. Bracard S, Ducrocq X, Mas JL, et al. Mechanical thrombectomy after intravenous alteplase versus alteplase alone after stroke (THRACE): a randomised controlled trial. Lancet Neurol,2016,15(11):1138-1147.
33. Sevick LK, Ghali S, Hill MD, et al. Systematic review of the cost and cost-effectiveness of rapid endovascular therapy for acute ischemic stroke. Stroke,2017,48(9):2519-2526.
34. Clinic C. Stroke. https://my.clevelandclinic.org/health/diseases/17519-stroke. Published 2018, Updated 2018, Oct 17 Accessed.
35. Lisabeth LD, Brown DL, Hughes R,et al. Acute stroke symptoms: comparing women and men. Stroke,2009,40(6):2031-2036.
36. Reeves M, Bhatt A, Jajou P, et al. Sex differences in the use of intravenous rt-PA thrombolysis treatment for acute ischemic stroke: a meta-analysis. Stroke,2009,40(5):1743-1749.
37. Barr J, McKinley S, O'Brien E, et al. Patient recognition of and response to symptoms of TIA or stroke. Neuroepidemiology,2006,26(3):168-175.
38. Centers for Disease Control,Prevention. Prehospital and hospital delays after stroke onset-United States, 2005-2006. MMWR Morb Mortal Wkly Rep,2007,56(19):474-478.
39. Cheung RT. Hong Kong patients' knowledge of stroke does not influence time-to-hospital presentation. J Clin Neurosci,2001,8(4):311-314.

40. Engelstein E, Margulies J, Jeret JS. Lack of t-PA use for acute ischemic stroke in a community hospital: high incidence of exclusion criteria. Am J Emerg Med,2000,18(3):257-260.
41. Foerch C, Misselwitz B, Humpich M, et al. Sex disparity in the access of elderly patients to acute stroke care. Stroke,2007,38(7):2123-2126.
42. Jungehulsing GJ, Rossnagel K, Nolte CH, et al. Emergency department delays in acute stroke-analysis of time between ED arrival and imaging. Eur J Neurol,2006,13(3):225-232.
43. Mandelzweig L, Goldbourt U, Boyko V, et al. Perceptual, social, and behavioral factors associated with delays in seeking medical care in patients with symptoms of acute stroke. Stroke,2006,37(5):1248-1253.
44. Menon SC, Pandey DK, Morgenstern LB. Critical factors determining access to acute stroke care. Neurology,1998,51(2):427-432.
45. Rose KM, Rosamond WD, Huston SL,et al. Predictors of time from hospital arrival to initial brain-imaging among suspected stroke patients: the North Carolina Collaborative Stroke Registry. Stroke,2008,39(12):3262-3267.
46. Yu RF, San Jose MC, Manzanilla BM,et al. Sources and reasons for delays in the care of acute stroke patients. J Neurol Sci,2002,199(1-2):49-54.
47. Chong J, Sacco RL. Risk factors for stroke, assessing risk, and the mass and high-risk approaches for stroke prevention//Gorelick PB. Continuum: Stroke Prevention. Hagerstwon, Maryland: Lippincott Williams and Wilkins,2005.
48. Johnston SC, Mendis S, Mathers CD. Global variation in stroke burden and mortality: estimates from monitoring, surveillance, and modelling. Lancet Neurol,2009,8(4):345-354.
49. Feigin VL, Norrving B, Mensah GA. Global Burden of Stroke. Circ Res,2017,120(3):439-448.
50. Gorelick PB. The global burden of stroke: persistent and disabling. Lancet Neurol,2019,18(5):417-418.
51. Katan M, Luft A. Global Burden of Stroke. Semin Neurol, 2018,38(2):208-211.
52. Goyal N, Tsivgoulis G, Malhotra K, et al. Medical management vs mechanical thrombectomy for mild strokes: an international multicenter study and systematic review and meta-analysis. JAMA Neurol, 2020,77(1):16-24.
53. Griessenauer CJ, Medin C, Maingard J, et al. Endovascular mechanical thrombectomy in large-vessel occlusion ischemic stroke presenting with low national institutes of health stroke scale: systematic review and meta-analysis. World Neurosurg,2018,110:263-269.
54. Heldner MR, Hsieh K, Broeg-Morvay A, et al. Clinical prediction of large vessel occlusion in

anterior circulation stroke: mission impossible? J Neurol,2016,263(8):1633-1640.

55. Li H, Zhang Y, Zhang L, et al. Endovascular treatment of acute ischemic stroke due to intracranial atherosclerotic large vessel occlusion : a systematic review. Clin Neuroradiol, 2020,30:777–787.

56. The Joint Commission. Specifications manual for joint commission national quality measures (v2018B1). https://manual.jointcommission.org/releases/TJC2018B1/DataElem0771.html. Published 2018. Accessed.

57. Dozois A, Hampton L, Kingston CW, et al. Plumber study prevalence of large vessel occlusion strokes in mecklenburg county emergency response. Stroke,2017,48(12):3397-3399.

58. Malhotra K, Gornbein J, Saver JL. Ischemic strokes due to large-vessel occlusions contribute disproportionately to stroke-related dependence and death: a review. Front Neurol,2017,8:651.

59. Rai AT, Seldon AE, Boo S, et al. A population-based incidence of acute large vessel occlusions and thrombectomy eligible patients indicates significant potential for growth of endovascular stroke therapy in the USA. J Neurointerv Surg,2017,9(8):722-726.

60. Smith WS, Lev MH, English JD, et al. Significance of large vessel intracranial occlusion causing acute ischemic stroke and TIA. Stroke,2009,40(12):3834-3840.

61. Rennert RC, Wali AR, Steinberg JA, et al. Epidemiology, natural history, and clinical presentation of large vessel ischemic stroke. Neurosurgery,2019,85(suppl 1):S4-S8.

62. Fink JN, Selim MH, Kumar S, et al. Insular cortex infarction in acute middle cerebral artery territory stroke: predictor of stroke severity and vascular lesion. Arch Neurol,2005,62(7):1081-1085.

63. Kodumuri N, Sebastian R, Davis C, et al. The association of insular stroke with lesion volume. Neuroimage Clin,2016,11:41-45.

64. Cooray C, Fekete K, Mikulik R, et al. Threshold for NIH stroke scale in predicting vessel occlusion and functional outcome after stroke thrombolysis. Int J Stroke,2015,10(6):822-829.

65. Heldner MR, Zubler C, Mattle HP, et al. National Institutes of Health stroke scale score and vessel occlusion in 2152 patients with acute ischemic stroke. Stroke,2013,44(4):1153-1157.

66. Al Kasab S, Holmstedt CA, Jauch EC,et al. Acute ischemic stroke due to large vessel occlusion. Emerg Med Rep,2018,39(2):13-22.

67. Brouns R, de Deyn PP. The complexity of neurobiological processes in acute ischemic stroke. Clin Neurol Neurosurg,2009,111(6):483-495.

68. Bansal S, Sangha KS, Khatri P. Drug treatment of acute ischemic stroke. Am J Cardiovasc

Drugs. 2013;13(1):57-69.

69. Bruno A, Biller J, Adams HP, et al. Acute blood glucose level and outcome from ischemic stroke,trial of org 10172 in acute stroke treatment (TOAST) investigators. Neurology,1999,52(2):280-284.

70. Catanese L, Tarsia J, Fisher M. Acute ischemic stroke therapy overview. Circ Res,2017,120(3):541-558.

71. de Rio-Espinola A, Fernandez-Cadenas I, Giralt D, et al. A predictive clinical-genetic model of tissue plasminogen activator response in acute ischemic stroke. Ann Neurol,2012,72(5):716-729.

72. Fernandez-Cadenas I, Del Rio-Espinola A, Giralt D, et al. IL1B and VWF variants are associated with fibrinolytic early recanalization in patients with ischemic stroke. Stroke,2012,43(10):2659-2665.

73. Mehta RH, Cox M, Smith EE, et al. Race/Ethnic differences in the risk of hemorrhagic complications among patients with ischemic stroke receiving thrombolytic therapy. Stroke,2014,45(8):2263-2269.

74. Savitz SI, Schlaug G, Caplan L, et al. Arterial occlusive lesions recanalize more frequently in women than in men after intravenous tissue plasminogen activator administration for acute stroke. Stroke, 2005,36(7):1447-1451.

75. Emberson J, Lees KR, Lyden P, et al. Effect of treatment delay, age, and stroke severity on the effects of intravenous thrombolysis with alteplase for acute ischaemic stroke: a meta-analysis of individual patient data from randomised trials. Lancet,2014,384(9958):1929-1935.

76. Riedel CH, Zimmermann P, Jensen-Kondering U, et al. The importance of size: successful recanalization by intravenous thrombolysis in acute anterior stroke depends on thrombus length. Stroke,2011,42(6):1775-1777.

77. de Zoppo GJ, Higashida RT, Furlan AJ, et al. PROACT: a phase II randomized trial of recombinant pro-urokinase by direct arterial delivery in acute middle cerebral artery stroke. PROACT Investigators. Prolyse in Acute Cerebral Thromboembolism. Stroke,1998,29(1):4-11.

78. Furlan A, Higashida R, Wechsler L, et al. Intra-arterial prourokinase for acute ischemic stroke. The PROACT II study: a randomized controlled trial. Prolyse in Acute Cerebral Thromboembolism. JAMA,1999,282(21):2003-2011.

79. National Institute of Neurological D, Stroke rt PASSG. Tissue plasminogen activator for acute ischemic stroke. N Engl J Med,1995,333(24):1581-1587.

80. Mechanical thrombectomy devices for acute ischaemic stroke. United Kingdom: National Institute for Health and Care Excellence,2018.
81. Hu YC, Stiefel MF. Force and aspiration analysis of the ADAPT technique in acute ischemic stroke treatment. J Neurointerv Surg,2016,8(3):244-246.
82. Group GBDNDC. Global, regional, and national burden of neurological disorders during 1990-2015: a systematic analysis for the global burden of disease study 2015. Lancet Neurol,2017,16(11):877-897.
83. Global Burden of Disease Study 2016. Global burden of disease study 2016 (GBD 2016) results.http://ghdx.healthdata.org/gbd-results-tool. Accessed 21 January 2020, 2020.
84. Krishnamurthi RV, Feigin VL, Forouzanfar MH, et al. Global and regional burden of first-ever ischaemic and haemorrhagic stroke during 1990-2010: findings from the global burden of disease study 2010. Lancet Glob Health,2013,1(5):e259-281.
85. Yang Q, Tong X, Schieb L, et al. Vital Signs: recent trends in stroke death rates — United States, 2000–2015. Morbidity and Mortality Weekly Report,2017,66(35):933-939.
86. Lozano R, Naghavi M, Foreman K, et al. Global and regional mortality from 235 causes of death for 20 age groups in 1990 and 2010: a systematic analysis for the global burden of disease study 2010. Lancet,2012,380(9859):2095-2128.
87. Boehme AK, Esenwa C, Elkind MS. Stroke risk factors, genetics, and prevention. Circ Res,2017,120(3):472-495.
88. O'Donnell MJ, Chin SL, Rangarajan S, et al. Global and regional effects of potentially modifiable risk factors associated with acute stroke in 32 countries (INTERSTROKE): a case-control study. Lancet,2016,388(10046):761-775.
89. Larsson SC, Wallin A, Wolk A, et al. Differing association of alcohol consumption with different stroke types: a systematic review and meta-analysis. BMC Med,2016,14(1):178.
90. Suk SH, Sacco RL, Boden-Albala B, et al. Abdominal obesity and risk of ischemic stroke: the northern manhattan stroke study. Stroke,2003,34(7):1586-1592.
91. Zhang X, Shu L, Si C, et al. Dietary patterns and risk of stroke in adults: a systematic review and meta-analysis of prospective cohort studies. J Stroke Cerebrovasc Dis,2015,24(10):2173-2182.
92. Boehme C, Toell T, Mayer L, et al. The dimension of preventable stroke in a large representative patient cohort. Neurology,2019,93(23):e2121-e2132.
93. Hachinski V, Donnan GA, Gorelick PB, et al. Stroke: working toward a prioritized world

agenda. Stroke,2010,41(6):1084-1099.

94. Pistoia F, Sacco S, Degan D,et al. Hypertension and stroke: epidemiological aspects and clinical evaluation. High Blood Press Cardiovasc Prev,2016,23(1):9-18.

95. Weiss J, Freeman M, Low A, et al. Benefits and harms of intensive blood pressure treatment in adults aged 60 years or older: a systematic review and meta-analysis. Ann Intern Med,2017,166(6):419-429.

96. Benjamin EJ, Virani SS, Callaway CW, et al. Heart disease and stroke statistics-2018 update: a report from the american heart association. Circulation,2018,137(12):e67-e492.

97. Benjamin EJ, Muntner P, Alonso A, et al. Heart disease and stroke statistics-2019 update: a report from the american heart association. Circulation,2019,139(10):e56-e528.

98. Law MR, Morris JK, Wald NJ. Use of blood pressure lowering drugs in the prevention of cardiovascular disease: meta-analysis of 147 randomised trials in the context of expectations from prospective epidemiological studies. BMJ,2009,338:b1665.

99. Lackland DT, Carey RM, Conforto AB, et al. Implications of recent clinical trials and hypertension guidelines on stroke and future cerebrovascular research. Stroke,2018,49(3):772-779.

100. Lau LH, Lew J, Borschmann K,et al. Prevalence of diabetes and its effects on stroke outcomes: a meta-analysis and literature review. J Diabetes Investig,2019,10(3):780-792.

101. Huxley R, Barzi F, Woodward M. Excess risk of fatal coronary heart disease associated with diabetes in men and women: meta-analysis of 37 prospective cohort studies. BMJ,2006,332(7533):73-78.

102. Peters SA, Huxley RR, Woodward M. Diabetes as a risk factor for stroke in women compared with men: a systematic review and meta-analysis of 64 cohorts, including 775,385 individuals and 12,539 strokes. Lancet,2014,383(9933):1973-1980.

103. Emerging Risk Factors Collaboration;,N Sarwar, P Gao, et al. Diabetes mellitus, fasting blood glucose concentration, and risk of vascular disease: a collaborative meta-analysis of 102 prospective studies. Lancet,2010,375(9733):2215-2222.

104. Banerjee C, Moon YP, Paik MC, et al. Duration of diabetes and risk of ischemic stroke: the Northern Manhattan Study. Stroke,2012,43(5):1212-1217.

105. Sui X, Lavie CJ, Hooker SP, et al. A prospective study of fasting plasma glucose and risk of stroke in asymptomatic men. Mayo Clin Proc,2011,86(11):1042-1049.

106. Kissela BM, Khoury J, Kleindorfer D, et al. Epidemiology of ischemic stroke in patients

with diabetes: the greater Cincinnati/Northern Kentucky Stroke Study. Diabetes Care,2005,28(2):355-359.

107. Roger VL, Go AS, Lloyd-Jones DM, et al. Heart disease and stroke statistics-2011 update: a report from the American Heart Association. Circulation,2011,123(4):e18-e209.

108. Ovbiagele B, Nguyen-Huynh MN. Stroke epidemiology: advancing our understanding of disease mechanism and therapy. Neurotherapeutics,2011,8(3):319-329.

109. Arboix A, Garcia-Eroles L, Massons J, et al. Acute stroke in very old people: clinical features and predictors of in-hospital mortality. J Am Geriatr Soc,2000,48(1):36-41.

110. Dennis MS, Burn JP, Sandercock PA, et al. Long-term survival after first-ever stroke: the Oxfordshire Community Stroke Project. Stroke,1993,24(6):796-800.

111. Di Carlo A, Lamassa M, Pracucci G, et al. Stroke in the very old : clinical presentation and determinants of 3-month functional outcome: A European perspective European BIOMED Study of Stroke Care Group. Stroke,1999,30(11):2313-2319.

112. Kammersgaard LP, Jorgensen HS, Reith J, et al. Short- and long-term prognosis for very old stroke patients:The Copenhagen Stroke Study. Age Ageing,2004,33(2):149-154.

113. Pohjasvaara T, Erkinjuntti T, Vataja R,et al. Comparison of stroke features and disability in daily life in patients with ischemic stroke aged 55 to 70 and 71 to 85 years. Stroke,1997,28(4):729-735.

114. Rojas JI, Zurru MC, Romano M,et al. Acute ischemic stroke and transient ischemic attack in the very old-risk factor profile and stroke subtype between patients older than 80 years and patients aged less than 80 years. Eur J Neurol,2007,14(8):895-899.

115. Krishnamurthi RV, Moran AE, Feigin VL, et al. Stroke prevalence, mortality and disability-adjusted life years in adults aged 20-64 years in 1990-2013: data from the global burden of disease 2013 study. Neuroepidemiology,2015,45(3):190-202.

116. Danaei G, Finucane MM, Lin JK, et al. National, regional, and global trends in systolic blood pressure since 1980: systematic analysis of health examination surveys and epidemiological studies with 786 country-years and 5.4 million participants. Lancet,2011,377(9765):568-577.

117. Norrving B, Kissela B. The global burden of stroke and need for a continuum of care. Neurology,2013,80(3 Suppl 2):S5-12.

118. de los Rios F, Kleindorfer DO, Khoury J, et al. Trends in substance abuse preceding stroke among young adults: a population-based study. Stroke,2012,43(12):3179-3183.

119. Zaridze D, Brennan P, Boreham J, et al. Alcohol and cause-specific mortality in Russia: a

retrospective case-control study of 48,557 adult deaths. Lancet,2009,373(9682):2201-2214.

120. Hu SS, Kong LZ, Gao RL, et al. Outline of the report on cardiovascular disease in China, 2010. Biomed Environ Sci,2012,25(3):251-256.

121. Jha P, Jacob B, Gajalakshmi V, et al. A nationally representative case-control study of smoking and death in India. N Engl J Med,2008,358(11):1137-1147.

122. Persky RW, Turtzo LC, McCullough LD. Stroke in women: disparities and outcomes. Curr Cardiol Rep,2010,12(1):6-13.

123. Roy-O'Reilly M, McCullough LD. Age and sex are critical factors in ischemic stroke pathology. Endocrinology,2018,159(8):3120-3131.

124. Appelros P, Nydevik I, Viitanen M. Poor outcome after first-ever stroke: predictors for death, dependency, and recurrent stroke within the first year. Stroke,2003,34(1):122-126.

125. Bots SH, Peters SAE, Woodward M. Sex differences in coronary heart disease and stroke mortality: a global assessment of the effect of ageing between 1980 and 2010. BMJ Glob Health,2017,2(2):e000298.

126. Collaborators GLRoS, Feigin VL, Nguyen G, et al. Global, regional, and country-specific lifetime risks of stroke, 1990 and 2016. N Engl J Med,2018,379(25):2429-2437.

127. Collaborators GBDCoD. Global, regional, and national age-sex specific mortality for 264 causes of death, 1980-2016: a systematic analysis for the Global Burden of Disease Study 2016. Lancet,2017,390(10100):1151-1210.

128. Zhu W, Churilov L, Campbell BC, et al. Does large vessel occlusion affect clinical outcome in stroke with mild neurologic deficits after intravenous thrombolysis? J Stroke Cerebrovasc Dis,2014,23(10):2888-2893.

129. Beumer D, Mulder MJHL, Saiedie G, et al. Occurrence of intracranial large vessel occlusion in consecutive, non-referred patients with acute ischemic stroke. Neurovasc Imaging,2016,2:11-16.

130. Hansen CK, Christensen A, Ovesen C, et al. Stroke severity and incidence of acute large vessel occlusions in patients with hyper-acute cerebral ischemia: results from a prospective cohort study based on CT-angiography (CTA). Int J Stroke,2015,10(3):336-342.

131. Miao Z, Huo X, Gao F, et al. Endovascular therapy for acute ischemic stroke trial (EAST): study protocol for a prospective, multicentre control trial in China. Stroke Vasc Neurol,2016,1(2):44-51.

132. Lakomkin N, Dhamoon M, Carroll K, et al. Prevalence of large vessel occlusion in patients

presenting with acute ischemic stroke: a 10-year systematic review of the literature. J Neurointerv Surg,2019,11(3):241-245.

133. Writing GM, Mozaffarian D, Benjamin EJ, et al. Heart disease and stroke statistics-2016 update: a report from the American Heart Association. Circulation,2016,133(4):e38-360.

134. Wang Y, Liao X, Zhao X, et al. Using recombinant tissue plasminogen activator to treat acute ischemic stroke in China: analysis of the results from the Chinese National Stroke Registry (CNSR). Stroke,2011,42(6):1658-1664.

135. Tsang ACO, You J, Li LF, et al. Burden of large vessel occlusion stroke and the service gap of thrombectomy: a population-based study using a territory-wide public hospital system registry. Int J Stroke,2020,15(1):69-74.

136. Institute for Health Metrics and Evaluation.Measuring what matters. University of Washington. Published 2019.

137. Takashima N, Arima H, Kita Y, et al. Incidence, management and short-term outcome of stroke in a general population of 1.4 million japanese- shiga stroke registry. Circ J,2017,81(11):1636-1646.

138. El-Hajj M, Salameh P, Rachidi S,et al. The epidemiology of stroke in the Middle East. Eur Stroke J,2016,1(3):180-198.

139. Alahmari K, Paul SS. Prevalence of stroke in kingdom of Saudi Arabia – through a physiotherapist diary. Mediterr J Soc Sci,2016,7:228-233.

140. Al-Rajeh S, Larbi EB, Bademosi O, et al. Stroke register: experience from the eastern province of Saudi Arabia. Cerebrovasc Dis,1998,8(2):86-89.

141. Al-Senani F, Al-Johani M, Salawati M, et al. A national economic and clinical model for ischemic stroke care development in Saudi Arabia: a call for change. Int J Stroke,2019,14(8):835-842.

142. Alhazzani AA, Mahfouz AA, Abolyazid AY, et al. Study of stroke incidence in the aseer region, Southwestern Saudi Arabia. Int J Environ Res Public Health,2018,15(2)215-222.

143. Alanazy MH, Barakeh RB, Asiri A, et al. Practice patterns and barriers for intravenous thrombolysis: a survey of neurologists in Saudi Arabia. Neurol Res Int, https://doi.org/10.1155/2018/1695014.

144. Horton R, Das P. Indian health: the path from crisis to progress. Lancet,2011,377(9761):181-183.

145. Dalal P, Bhattacharjee M, Vairale J,et al. UN millennium development goals: Can we halt the

stroke epidemic in India? Ann Indian Acad Neurol,2007,10(3):130-136.

146. Kamalakannan S, Gudlavalleti ASV, Gudlavalleti VSM,et al. Incidence & prevalence of stroke in India:a systematic review. Indian J Med Res,2017,146(2):175-185.

147. Feigin VL, Lawes CM, Bennett DA,et al. Worldwide stroke incidence and early case fatality reported in 56 population-based studies: a systematic review. Lancet Neurol,2009,8(4):355-369.

148. Bennett DA, Krishnamurthi RV, Barker-Collo S, et al. The global burden of ischemic stroke: findings of the GBD 2010 study. Glob Heart,2014,9(1):107-112.

149. Huded V, Nair RR, de Souza R, et al. Endovascular treatment of acute ischemic stroke: an Indian experience from a tertiary care center. Neurol India,2014,62(3):276-279.

150. Truelsen T, Hansen K, Andersen G, et al. Acute endovascular reperfusion treatment in patients with ischaemic stroke and large-vessel occlusion (Denmark 2011-2017). Eur J Neurol, 2019,26(8):1044-1050.

151. von Kummer R, Allen KL, Holle R, et al. Acute stroke: usefulness of early CT findings before thrombolytic therapy. Radiology,1997,205(2):327-333.

152. Lees KR, Bluhmki E, von Kummer R, et al. Time to treatment with intravenous alteplase and outcome in stroke: an updated pooled analysis of ECASS, ATLANTIS, NINDS, and EPITHET trials. Lancet,2010,375(9727):1695-1703.

153. Kwiatkowski TG, Libman RB, Frankel M, et al. Effects of tissue plasminogen activator for acute ischemic stroke at one year. National Institute of Neurological Disorders and Stroke Recombinant Tissue Plasminogen Activator Stroke Study Group. N Engl J Med,1999,340(23):1781-1787.

154. Hacke W, Kaste M, Bluhmki E, et al. Thrombolysis with alteplase 3 to 4.5 hours after acute ischemic stroke. N Engl J Med,2008,359(13):1317-1329.

155. Balami JS, Hadley G, Sutherland BA,et al. The exact science of stroke thrombolysis and the quiet art of patient selection. Brain,2013,136(Pt 12):3528-3553.

156. Paciaroni M, Inzitari D, Agnelli G, et al. Intravenous thrombolysis or endovascular therapy for acute ischemic stroke associated with cervical internal carotid artery occlusion: the ICARO-3 study. J Neurol,2015,262(2):459-468.

157. Yoo AJ, Pulli B, Gonzalez RG. Imaging-based treatment selection for intravenous and intra-arterial stroke therapies: a comprehensive review. Expert Rev Cardiovasc Ther,2011,9(7):857-876.

158. Fisher M, Albers GW. Advanced imaging to extend the therapeutic time window of acute ischemic stroke. Ann Neurol,2013,73(1):4-9.

159. Duffis EJ, Al-Qudah Z, Prestigiacomo CJ,et al. Advanced neuroimaging in acute ischemic stroke: extending the time window for treatment. Neurosurg Focus,2011,30(6):E5.

160. Sandhu GS, Sunshine JL. Advanced neuroimaging to guide acute stroke therapy. Curr Cardiol Rep,2012,14(6):741-753.

161. Medlin F, Amiguet M, Vanacker P,et al. Influence of arterial occlusion on outcome after intravenous thrombolysis for acute ischemic stroke. Stroke,2015,46(1):126-131.

162. Hong JH, Sohn SI, Kang J, et al. Endovascular treatment in patients with persistent internal carotid artery occlusion after intravenous tissue plasminogen activator: a clinical effectiveness study. Cerebrovasc Dis,2016,42(5-6):387-394.

163. Paciaroni M, Balucani C, Agnelli G, et al. Systemic thrombolysis in patients with acute ischemic stroke and internal carotid artery occlusion: the ICARO study. Stroke,2012,43(1):125-130.

164. Saqqur M, Tsivgoulis G, Molina CA, et al. Residual flow at the site of intracranial occlusion on transcranial doppler predicts response to intravenous thrombolysis: a multi-center study. Cerebrovasc Dis,2009,27(1):5-12.

165. Saqqur M, Uchino K, Demchuk AM, et al. Site of arterial occlusion identified by transcranial Doppler predicts the response to intravenous thrombolysis for stroke. Stroke,2007,38(3):948-954.

166. Rubiera M, Ribo M, Delgado-Mederos R, et al. Tandem internal carotid artery/middle cerebral artery occlusion: an independent predictor of poor outcome after systemic thrombolysis. Stroke,2006,37(9):2301-2305.

167. Khandelwal P, Yavagal DR, Sacco RL. Acute Ischemic stroke intervention. J Am Coll Cardiol,2016,67(22):2631-2644.

168. Liu X. Beyond the time window of intravenous thrombolysis: standing by or by stenting? Interv Neurol,2012,1(1):3-15.

169. Wolpert SM, Bruckmann H, Greenlee R,et al. Neuroradiologic evaluation of patients with acute stroke treated with recombinant tissue plasminogen activator. The rt-PA Acute Stroke Study Group. AJNR Am J Neuroradiol,1993,14(1):3-13.

170. Stroke, Cerebrovascular Accident. World Health Organization. http://www.emro.who.int/health-topics/stroke-cerebrovascular-accident/index.html. Published 2019.

171. Demand for Neurovascular Thrombectomy Devices to Surge on Account of Growing Incidences of Acute Ischemic Stroke. BioSpace. https://www.biospace.com/article/demand-for-neurovascular-thrombectomy-devices-to-surge-on-account-of-growing-incidences-of-acute-ischemic-stroke/. Published 2019.

172. Li YY. Stroke devices medtech 360 market analysis US 2018. 2018.

173. Zaidat OO, Lazzaro M, McGinley E, et al. Demand-supply of neurointerventionalists for endovascular ischemic stroke therapy. Neurology, 2012,79(13 Suppl 1):S35-41.

174. Fiorella D, Cloft H. Demand-supply of neurointerventionalists for endovascular ischemic stroke therapy. Neurology,2013,81(3):305.

175. Gupta R, Horev A, Nguyen T, et al. Higher volume endovascular stroke centers have faster times to treatment, higher reperfusion rates and higher rates of good clinical outcomes. J Neurointerv Surg,2013,5(4):294-297.

176. Avasarala J, Wesley K. Optimization of acute stroke care in the emergency department: a call for better utilization of healthcare resources amid growing shortage of neurologists in the United States. CNS Spectr, 2018,23(4):248-250.

177. Sigsbee B, Bernat JL. Physician burnout: A neurologic crisis. Neurology,2014,83(24):2302-2306.

178. Dall TM, Storm MV, Chakrabarti R, et al. Supply and demand analysis of the current and future US neurology workforce. Neurology,2013,81(5):470-478.

179. Vanacker P, Lambrou D, Eskandari A,et al. Eligibility and predictors for acute revascularization procedures in a stroke center. Stroke,2016,47(7):1844-1849.

180. Tawil SE, Cheripelli B, Huang X, et al. How many stroke patients might be eligible for mechanical thrombectomy? Eur Stroke J,2016,1(4):264-271.

181. Wahlgren N, Moreira T, Michel P, et al. Mechanical thrombectomy in acute ischemic stroke: consensus statement by ESO-Karolinska Stroke Update 2014/2015, supported by ESO, ESMINT, ESNR and EAN. Int J Stroke,2016,11(1):134-147.

182. Kuntze Soderqvist A, Andersson T, Ahmed N,et al. Thrombectomy in acute ischemic stroke: estimations of increasing demands. J Neurointerv Surg,2017,9(9):830-833.

183. Wanted: More interventionalists. NeuroNews International. https://neuronewsinternational.com/wanted-more-interventionalists/. Published 2017.

184. Urimubenshi G, Cadilhac DA, Kagwiza JN,et al. Stroke care in Africa: a systematic review of the literature. Int J Stroke,2018,13(8):797-805.

185. Al-Senani F, Salawati M, AlJohani M,et al. Workforce requirements for comprehensive ischaemic stroke care in a developing country: the case of Saudi Arabia. Hum Resour Health,2019,17(1):90.

186. Fujiwara K, Osanai T, Kobayashi E, et al. Accessibility to tertiary stroke centers in Hokkaido, Japan: Use of novel metrics to assess acute stroke care quality. J Stroke Cerebrovasc Dis,2018,27(1):177-184.

187. Brinjikji W, Starke RM, Murad MH, et al. Impact of balloon guide catheter on technical and clinical outcomes: a systematic review and meta-analysis. J Neurointerv Surg,2018,10(4):335-339.

188. Goyal M, Menon BK, van Zwam WH, et al. Endovascular thrombectomy after large-vessel ischaemic stroke: a meta-analysis of individual patient data from five randomised trials. Lancet,2016,387(10029):1723-1731.

189. Minnerup J, Wersching H, Teuber A, et al. Outcome after thrombectomy and intravenous thrombolysis in patients with acute ischemic stroke: a prospective observational study. Stroke,2016,47(6):1584-1592.

190. Mellon L, Doyle F, Williams D,et al. Patient behaviour at the time of stroke onset: a cross-sectional survey of patient response to stroke symptoms. Emerg Med J,2016,33(6):396-402.

191. Glober NK, Sporer KA, Guluma KZ, et al. Acute stroke: current evidence-based recommendations for prehospital care. West J Emerg Med,2016,17(2):104-128.

192. Elizabeth K,Powell HGC, Natalie PK. Acute Stroke: from prehospital care to in-hospital management. Journal of Emergency Medical Services,2018,43(5):182-184.

193. Waqas M, Vakharia K, Munich SA, et al. Initial emergency room triage of acute ischemic stroke. Neurosurgery,2019,85(Suppl 1):s38-s46.

194. Chang P, Prabhakaran S. Recent advances in the management of acute ischemic stroke. F1000Res. 2017,6.

195. Hasan TF, Rabinstein AA, Middlebrooks EH, et al. Diagnosis and management of acute ischemic stroke. Mayo Clinic Proceedings, 2018,93(4):523-538.

196. Zweifler RM. Initial assessment and triage of the stroke patient. Prog Cardiovasc Dis,2017,59(6):527-533.

197. Mayo Clinic Staff. Stroke. Mayo Foundation for Medical Education and Research (MFMER). https://www.mayoclinic.org/diseases-conditions/stroke/diagnosis-treatment/drc-20350119. Accessed December 21,2019.

198. Azzam EI, Jay-Gerin JP, Pain D. Ionizing radiation-induced metabolic oxidative stress and prolonged cell injury. Cancer Lett,2012,327(1-2):48-60.

199. Powers WJ, Rabinstein AA, Ackerson T, et al. 2018 Guidelines for the early management of patients with acute ischemic stroke: a guideline for healthcare professionals from the American Heart Association/American Stroke Association. Stroke,2018,49(3):e46-e110.

200. Powers WJ, Derdeyn CP, Biller J, et al. 2015 American Heart Association/American Stroke Association focused update of the 2013 guidelines for the early management of patients with acute ischemic stroke regarding endovascular treatment: a guideline for healthcare professionals from the American Heart Association/American Stroke Association. Stroke,2015,46(10):3020-3035.

201. Saver JL, Fonarow GC, Smith EE, et al. Time to treatment with intravenous tissue plasminogen activator and outcome from acute ischemic stroke. JAMA,2013,309(23):2480-2488.

202. Fanous AA, Siddiqui AH. Mechanical thrombectomy: stent retrievers *vs* aspiration catheters. Cor et vasa,2016,58(2):e193-203.

203. Lee W, Sitoh YY, Lim CC, et al. The MERCI Retrieval System for the management of acute ischaemic stroke-the NNI Singapore experience. Ann Acad Med Singapore,2009,38(9):749-755.

204. Alshekhlee A, Pandya DJ, English J, et al. Merci mechanical thrombectomy retriever for acute ischemic stroke therapy: literature review. Neurology,2012,79(13 Suppl 1):S126-134.

205. Jeong HS, Shin JW, Kwon HJ, et al. Cost benefits of rapid recanalization using intraarterial thrombectomy. Brain and behavior, 2017,7(10):e00830.

206. Mu F, Hurley D, Betts KA, et al. Real-world costs of ischemic stroke by discharge status. Current medical research and opinion,2017,33(2):371-378.

207. Rai AT, Crivera C, Kalsekar I, et al. Endovascular stroke therapy trends from 2011 to 2017 show significant improvement in clinical and economic outcomes. Stroke,2019,50(7):1902-1906.

208. Kunz WG, Hunink MG, Dimitriadis K, et al. Cost-effectiveness of endovascular therapy for acute ischemic stroke: a systematic review of the impact of patient age. Radiology,2018,288(2):518-526.

209. Mittmann N, Seung SJ, Hill MD, et al. Impact of disability status on ischemic stroke costs in Canada in the first year. Can J Neurol Sci, 2012,39(6):793-800.

210. Xie X, Lambrinos A, Chan B, et al. Mechanical thrombectomy in patients with acute ischemic stroke: a cost-utility analysis. CMAJ Open,2016,4(2):e316-325.

211. Koto PS, Hu SX, Virani K, et al. A cost-utility analysis of endovascular thrombectomy in a real-world setting. Can J Neurol Sci,2019,1-11.

212. Pizzo E, Dumba M, Lobotesis K. Cost-utility analysis of mechanical thrombectomy between 6 and 24 hours in acute ischemic stroke. Int J Stroke,2019,1747493019830587.

213. Ganesalingam J, Pizzo E, Morris S,et al. Cost-utility analysis of mechanical thrombectomy using stent retrievers in acute ischemic stroke. Stroke,2015,46(9):2591-2598.

214. Heggie R, Wu O, White P, et al. Mechanical thrombectomy in patients with acute ischemic stroke: a cost-effectiveness and value of implementation analysis. Int J Stroke,2019,1747493019879656.

215. Lobotesis K, Veltkamp R, Carpenter IH, et al. Cost-effectiveness of stent-retriever thrombectomy in combination with IV t-PA compared with IV t-PA alone for acute ischemic stroke in the UK. J Med Econ,2016,19(8):785-794.

216. Achit H, Soudant M, Hosseini K, et al. Cost-effectiveness of thrombectomy in patients with acute ischemic stroke: the THRACE randomized controlled trial. Stroke,2017,48(10):2843-2847.

217. Kabore N, Marnat G, Rouanet F, et al. Cost-effectiveness analysis of mechanical thrombectomy plus tissue-type plasminogen activator compared with tissue-type plasminogen activator alone for acute ischemic stroke in France. Rev Neurol (Paris),2019,175(4):252-260.

218. Steen CK, Andsberg G, Petersson J, et al. Long-term cost-effectiveness of thrombectomy for acute ischaemic stroke in real life: an analysis based on data from the Swedish Stroke Register (Riksstroke). International journal of stroke : official journal of the International Stroke Society, 2017,12(8):802-814.

219. Aronsson M, Persson J, Blomstrand C,et al. Cost-effectiveness of endovascular thrombectomy in patients with acute ischemic stroke. Neurology,2016,86(11):1053-1059.

220. Ruggeri M, Basile M, Zini A, et al. Cost-effectiveness analysis of mechanical thrombectomy with stent retriever in the treatment of acute ischemic stroke in Italy. J Med Econ,2018,21(9):902-911.

221. de Andres-Nogales F, Alvarez M, de Miquel MA, et al. Cost-effectiveness of mechanical thrombectomy using stent retriever after intravenous tissue plasminogen activator compared

with intravenous tissue plasminogen activator alone in the treatment of acute ischaemic stroke due to large vessel occlusion in Spain. Eur Stroke J,2017,2(3):272-284.

222. Arora N, Makino K, Tilden D,et al. Cost-effectiveness of mechanical thrombectomy for acute ischemic stroke: an Australian payer perspective. Journal of medical economics,2018,21(8):799-809.

223. Pan Y, Cai X, Huo X, et al. Cost-effectiveness of mechanical thrombectomy within 6 hours of acute ischaemic stroke in China. BMJ Open,2018,8(2):e018951.

224. Muir KW, Ford GA, Messow CM, et al. Endovascular therapy for acute ischaemic stroke: the pragmatic ischaemic stroke thrombectomy evaluation (PISTE) randomised, controlled trial. J Neurol Neurosurg Psychiatry,2017,88(1):38-44.

225. Flynn D, Francis R, Halvorsrud K, et al. Intra-arterial mechanical thrombectomy stent retrievers and aspiration devices in the treatment of acute ischaemic stroke: a systematic review and meta-analysis with trial sequential analysis. Eur Stroke J,2017,2(4):308-318.

226. Saver JL, Jahan R, Levy EI, et al. Solitaire flow restoration device versus the Merci Retriever in patients with acute ischaemic stroke (SWIFT): a randomised, parallel-group, non-inferiority trial. Lancet,2012,380(9849):1241-1249.

227. Mechanical thrombectomy for acute ischaemic stroke: An implementation guide for the UK. Oxford Academic Health Science Network,2019.

228. Boudour S, Barral M, Gory B, et al. A systematic review of economic evaluations on stent-retriever thrombectomy for acute ischemic stroke. J Neurol,2018,265(7):1511-1520.

229. Powers WJ, Rabinstein AA, Ackerson T, et al. Guidelines for the early management of patients with acute ischemic stroke: 2019 update to the 2018 guidelines for the early management of acute ischemic stroke: a guideline for healthcare professionals from the American Heart Association/American Stroke Association. Stroke,2019,50(12):e344-e418.

230. Adeoye O, Nystrom KV, Yavagal DR, et al. Recommendations for the establishment of stroke systems of care: a 2019 update. Stroke, 2019,50(7):e187-e210.

231. Ojike N, Ravenell J, Seixas A, et al. Racial disparity in stroke awareness in the US: an analysis of the 2014 national health interview survey. J Neurol Neurophysiol,2016,7(2).

232. Hassan AE, Kassel DH, Adil MM,et al. Are there disparities in thrombolytic treatment and mortality in acute ischemic stroke in the hispanic population living in border states versus nonborder states? J Vasc Interv Neurol,2016,9(2):1-4.

233. Ekundayo OJ, Saver JL, Fonarow GC, et al. Patterns of emergency medical services use and

its association with timely stroke treatment: findings from get with the guidelines-stroke. Circ Cardiovasc Qual Outcomes,2013,6(3):262-269.

234. Crocco TJ, Grotta JC, Jauch EC, et al. EMS management of acute stroke-prehospital triage (resource document to NAEMSP position statement). Prehosp Emerg Care, 2007,11(3):313-317.

235. Berglund A, Svensson L, Wahlgren N, et al. Face arm speech time test use in the prehospital setting, better in the ambulance than in the emergency medical communication center. Cerebrovasc Dis,2014,37(3):212-216.

236. De Luca A, Giorgi Rossi P, Villa GF, et al. The use of Cincinnati prehospital stroke scale during telephone dispatch interview increases the accuracy in identifying stroke and transient ischemic attack symptoms. BMC Health Serv Res,2013,13:513.

237. Bray JE, Martin J, Cooper G,et al. Paramedic identification of stroke: community validation of the melbourne ambulance stroke screen. Cerebrovasc Dis,2005,20(1):28-33.

238. Bray JE, Martin J, Cooper G, et al. An interventional study to improve paramedic diagnosis of stroke. Prehosp Emerg Care,2005,9(3):297-302.

239. Kidwell CS, Saver JL, Schubert GB, et al. Design and retrospective analysis of the Los Angeles Prehospital Stroke Screen (LAPSS). Prehosp Emerg Care,1998,2(4):267-273.

240. Kidwell CS, Starkman S, Eckstein M, et al. Identifying stroke in the field. Prospective validation of the Los Angeles prehospital stroke screen (LAPSS). Stroke,2000,31(1):71-76.

241. Navalkele D, Vahidy F, Kendrick S, et al. Vision, aphasia, neglect assessment for large vessel occlusion stroke. J Stroke Cerebrovasc Dis, 2020,29(1):104478.

242. Teleb MS, Ver Hage A, Carter J,et al. Stroke vision, aphasia, neglect (VAN) assessment-a novel emergent large vessel occlusion screening tool: pilot study and comparison with current clinical severity indices. J Neurointerv Surg,2017,9(2):122-126.

243. Ver Hage A, Teleb M, Smith E. An emergent large vessel occlusion screening protocol for acute stroke: a quality improvement initiative. J Neurosci Nurs,2018,50(2):68-73.

244. Lin CB, Peterson ED, Smith EE, et al. Emergency medical service hospital prenotification is associated with improved evaluation and treatment of acute ischemic stroke. Circ Cardiovasc Qual Outcomes,2012,5(4):514-522.

245. Lavine SD, Cockroft K, Hoh B, et al. Training guidelines for endovascular ischemic stroke intervention: an international multi-society consensus document. AJNR Am J Neuroradiol, 2016,37(4):e31-34.

246. Meyers PM, Schumacher HC, Alexander MJ, et al. Performance and training standards for endovascular ischemic stroke treatment. J Stroke Cerebrovasc Dis,2009,18(6):411-415.

247. Grigoryan M, Chaudhry SA, Hassan AE,et al. Neurointerventional procedural volume per hospital in United States: implications for comprehensive stroke center designation. Stroke,2012,43(5):1309-1314.

248. Goyal M, Jadhav AP, Bonafe A, et al. Analysis of workflow and time to treatment and the effects on outcome in endovascular treatment of acute ischemic stroke: results from the SWIFT PRIME randomized controlled trial. Radiology,2016,279(3):888-897.

249. Tahtali D, Bohmann F, Rostek P,et al. Setting up a stroke team algorithm and conducting simulation-based training in the emergency department - a practical guide. J Vis Exp,2017(119).

250. Tahtali D, Bohmann F, Kurka N, et al. Implementation of stroke teams and simulation training shortened process times in a regional stroke network-A network-wide prospective trial. PLoS One,2017,12(12):e0188231.

251. English JD, Yavagal DR, Gupta R, et al. Mechanical thrombectomy-ready comprehensive stroke center requirements and endovascular stroke systems of care: recommendations from the endovascular stroke standards committee of the society of vascular and interventional neurology (SVIN). Interv Neurol,2016,4(3-4):138-150.

252. Boogaarts HD, van Amerongen MJ, de Vries J, et al. Caseload as a factor for outcome in aneurysmal subarachnoid hemorrhage: a systematic review and meta-analysis. J Neurosurg,2014,120(3):605-611.

253. Demetriades D, Martin M, Salim A,et al. The effect of trauma center designation and trauma volume on outcome in specific severe injuries. Ann Surg, 2005,242(4):512-517.

254. McGrath PD, Wennberg DE, Dickens JD, et al. Relation between operator and hospital volume and outcomes following percutaneous coronary interventions in the era of the coronary stent. JAMA,2000,284(24):3139-3144.

255. Prabhakaran S, Fonarow GC, Smith EE, et al. Hospital case volume is associated with mortality in patients hospitalized with subarachnoid hemorrhage. Neurosurgery,2014,75(5):500-508.

256. Kollikowski AM, Amaya F, Stoll G,et al. Impact of landmark endovascular stroke trials on logistical performance measures: a before-and-after evaluation of real-world data from a regional stroke system of care. J Neurointerv Surg,2019,11(6):563-568.

257. McTaggart RA, Moldovan K, Oliver LA, et al. Door-in-Door-Out Time at primary stroke centers may predict outcome for emergent large vessel occlusion patients. Stroke,2018,49(12):2969-2974.

258. Ng FC, Low E, Andrew E, et al. Deconstruction of interhospital transfer workflow in large vessel occlusion: real-world data in the thrombectomy era. Stroke,2017,48(7):1976-1979.

259. Choi PMC, Tsoi AH, Pope AL, et al. Door-in-Door-Out Time of 60 minutes for stroke with emergent large vessel occlusion at a primary stroke center. Stroke,2019,50(10):2829-2834.

260. Venema E, Lingsma HF, Chalos V, et al. Personalized prehospital triage in acute ischemic stroke. Stroke,2019,50(2):313-320.

261. Mokin M, Gupta R, Guerrero WR,et al. ASPECTS decay during inter-facility transfer in patients with large vessel occlusion strokes. J Neurointerv Surg,2017,9(5):442-444.

262. Froehler MT, Saver JL, Zaidat OO, et al. Interhospital transfer before thrombectomy is associated with delayed treatment and worse outcome in the STRATIS Registry (systematic evaluation of patients treated with neurothrombectomy devices for acute ischemic stroke). Circulation,2017,136(24):2311-2321.

263. Venema E, Groot AE, Lingsma HF, et al. Effect of interhospital transfer on endovascular treatment for acute ischemic stroke. Stroke,2019,50(4):923-930.

264. Jayaraman MV, Hemendinger ML, Baird GL, et al. Field triage for endovascular stroke therapy: a population-based comparison. J Neurointerv Surg,2019.

265. Seker F, Bonekamp S, Rode S,et al. Direct admission *vs* secondary transfer to a comprehensive stroke center for thrombectomy : retrospective analysis of a regional stroke registry with 2797 patients. Clin Neuroradiol,2019.

266. Grotta JC. Interhospital transfer of stroke patients for endovascular treatment. Circulation,2019,139(13):1578-1580.

267. George BP, Pieters TA, Zammit CG,et al. Trends in interhospital transfers and mechanical thrombectomy for United States acute ischemic stroke inpatients. J Stroke Cerebrovasc Dis,2019,28(4):980-987.

268. Sablot D, Dumitrana A, Leibinger F, et al. Futile inter-hospital transfer for mechanical thrombectomy in a semi-rural context: analysis of a 6-year prospective registry. J Neurointerv Surg,2019,11(6):539-544.

269. Morey JR, Dangayach NS, Shoirah H, et al. Major causes for not performing endovascular therapy following inter-hospital transfer in a complex urban setting. Cerebrovasc Dis,2019:1-

6.

270. Asif KS, Lazzaro MA, Zaidat O. Identifying delays to mechanical thrombectomy for acute stroke: onset to door and door to clot times. J Neurointerv Surg,2014,6(7):505-510.

271. Al Kasab S, Almallouhi E, Harvey J, et al. Door in door out and transportation times in 2 telestroke networks. Neurol Clin Pract,2019,9(1):41-47.

272. Sablot D, Farouil G, Laverdure A,et al. Shortening time to reperfusion after transfer from a primary to a comprehensive stroke center. Neurol Clin Pract,2019,9(5):417-423.

273. McTaggart RA, Yaghi S, Baird G,et al. Decreasing procedure times with a standardized approach to ELVO cases. J Neurointerv Surg,2017,9(1):2-5.

274. Wei D, Oxley TJ, Nistal DA, et al. Mobile interventional stroke teams lead to faster treatment times for thrombectomy in large vessel occlusion. Stroke,2017,48(12):3295-3300.

275. Leira EC, Stilley JD, Schnell T,et al. Helicopter transportation in the era of thrombectomy: the next frontier for acute stroke treatment and research. Eur Stroke J,2016,1(3):171-179.

276. Vaughan SM, Limaye K, Samaniego EA, et al. Disparities in Inter-hospital helicopter transportation for hispanics by geographic region: a threat to fairness in the era of thrombectomy. J Stroke Cerebrovasc Dis,2019,28(3):550-556.